Perinatal Neurology
and Neurosurgery

Perinatal Neurology and Neurosurgery

Edited by

Richard A. Thompson, M.D.
John R. Green, M.D., F.A.C.S.
Stanley D. Johnsen, M.D.

Barrow Neurological Institute
St. Joseph's Hospital and Medical Center
Phoenix, Arizona

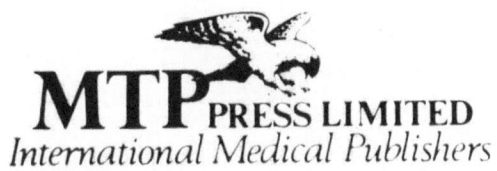

MTP PRESS LIMITED
International Medical Publishers

Published in the UK and Europe by
MTP Press Limited
Falcon House
Lancaster, England

Published in the US by
SPECTRUM PUBLICATIONS, INC.
175-20 Wexford Terrace
Jamaica, NY   11432

ISBN-13: 978-94-011-7297-4   e-ISBN-13: 978-94-011-7295-0
DOI: 10.1007/978-94-011-7295-0

Contributors

Diane S. Babcock, M.D. • Associate Professor of Radiology and Assistant Professor of Pediatrics, University of Cincinnati College of Medicine, Children's Hospital Medical Center, Cincinnati, Ohio

Alfred Brann, Jr., M.D. • Professor, Pediatrics, Gynecology and Obstetrics; Director, Division of Neonatal and Perinatal Medicine, Emory University School of Medicine, Atlanta, Georgia

Jan Goddard-Finegold, M.D. • Assistant Professor, Pediatrics and Pathology, Baylor College of Medicine; Texas Children's Hospital, Houston, Texas

Patricia Goldman-Rakic, Ph.D. • Professor, Neuroscience, Section of Neuroanatomy, Yale University School of Medicine, New Haven, Connecticut

Gary W. Goldstein, M.D. • Professor, Pediatrics and Neurology; Director, Section of Pediatric Neurology, University of Michigan School of Medicine, Ann Arbor, Michigan

Hector E. James, M.D. • Associate Professor, Neurosurgery and Pediatrics, University of California Medical Center, San Diego, California

Allen Merritt, M.D. • University of California, San Diego, California

H. Belton P. Meyer, M.D. • Co-Director, Division of Reproductive Medicine, St. Joseph's Hospital and Medical Center, Phoenix, Arizona

Pasko Rakic, M.D., Sc.D. • Professor, Neuroscience; Chairman, Section of Neuroanatomy, Yale University School of Medicine, New Haven, Connecticut

Elsa J. Sell, M.D. • Associate Professor, Pediatrics; Clinical Head, Section of Perinatal and Nutritional Sciences; Director, Newborn Follow-up Clinic, University of Arizona, Health Sciences Center, Tucson, Arizona

Daniel C. Shannon, M.D. • Associate Professor, Pediatrics, Harvard-MIT, Division of Health Sciences and Technology; Director, Pediatric Pulmonary Unit, Massachusetts General Hospital, Boston, Massachusetts

James J. Stockard, M.D., Ph.D. • Watson Clinic, Lakeland Medical Center, Lakeland, Florida; Associate Professor, Department of Neurology, University of South Florida Medical Center, Tampa, Florida

Janet E. Stockard, B.A. • Departments of Communicology and Pediatrics, University of South Florida, Tampa, Florida

Robert C. Vannucci, M.D. • Associate Professor, Pediatrics and Neurology, Cornell University Medical College; Chief, Pediatric Neurology, New York Hospital, New York, New York

Preface

This volume represents a collection of topics presented at the Tenth Annual Symposium of the Barrow Neurological Institute. No attempt is made to be comprehensive but rather an attempt is made to give adequate attention to the major important topics in this field. Neurodevelopmental biology, pathophysiology, and laboratory evaluation are discussed. Subjects include hypoxic ischemia, intraventricular hemorrhage, fetal neurosurgery, surgery of hydrocephalus, problems of apnea, ultrasound and CT imaging techniques, electrodiagnosis and ethical and economic issues. This volume will be of interest to neurologists and neurosurgeons in general, and especially to pediatric neurologists and neurosurgeons, and perinatologists.

Richard A. Thompson, M.D.
John R. Green, M.D.
Stanley D. Johnsen, M.D.

Contents

Acknowledgments

We are indebted to the internationally recognized authors who have contributed to this volume and to the excellent Symposium upon which it was based, and to the Barrow Neurological Symposium Committee of Richard A. Thompson, M. D., Chairman; Carlos A. Carrion, M.D.; Charles L. Echols, Jr., M.D.; Lisa Wilkinson Fannin, M.D.; John R. Green, M.D.; William B. Helme, M.D.; John A. Hodak, M.D.; Stanley D. Johnsen, M.D.; Edward H. Lipson, M.D.; Daniel A. Pollen, M.D.; Marilyn M. Ricci, R.N.; John D. Waggener, M.D.; and Joseph C. White, Jr., M.D.

CHAPTER 1

Use of Fetal Neurosurgery for Experimental Studies of Structural and Functional Brain Development in Nonhuman Primates

Pasko Rakic, M.D., Sc.D., Patricia S. Goldman-Rakic, Ph.D.

A major obstacle to the experimental analysis of mammalian brain development is its inaccessibility in the well protected environment of the uterus. The problem of access is particularly great in developmental studies of the primate brain, which achieves a high degree of maturity *in utero* and in which many significant cellular events and critical developmental periods occur before the time of birth. Thus, it is perhaps not surprising that until recently no detailed information was available on the prenatal development of brain in any primate species. Indeed, the only sources of information on this subject were anatomical studies carried out on postmortem fixed human fetal tissue. However, during the past decade the techniques of prenatal neurosurgery have been refined to a point that prenatal manipulations have become an important part of the variety of experimental approaches to the study of brain development in mammals. In a short period of time, this approach has provided a new body of data that is of considerable practical and conceptual importance for understanding neurogenesis in mammals and indirectly that of the human fetal brain. Significantly, these procedures

Perinatal Neurology and Neurosurgery. Edited by R. A. Thompson, J. R. Green, and S. D. Johnsen. Copyright © 1985 by Spectrum Publications, Inc.

present little danger to the mother and can be performed with a high expectancy of survival for the operated fetuses. It should be emphasized that the type of experimental neurosurgery performed in animals is usually considerably more extensive than any correctional or diagnostic procedure that has ever been attempted on or contemplated for human fetuses *in utero*. To our knowledge, fetal surgery in humans has been limited to the implantation of shunts for the treatment of hydrocephalus or for procedures intended to correct urinary tract obstruction [1].

In the present article, we limit ourselves to a discussion of experimental neurosurgery in rhesus monkeys. We first review some historical aspects of fetal neurosurgery in large mammals including primates. Second, we describe the general management and basic techniques of neurosurgery on rhesus monkey fetuses in our laboratories. Finally, we briefly discuss some present and possible future uses and benefits of experimental manipulation of the fetal brain in the field of developmental neurobiology. Perhaps it is equally important to underscore what is not covered in our presentation: we do not present our experience as advice or encouragement for diagnostic or therapeutic procedures in humans. The procedures and techniques described are based mostly on our own experience using prenatal neurosurgery in the past decade, and, as a consequence, our emphasis is mostly, if not exclusively, on the problems encountered in dealing with pregnant rhesus monkeys, their fetuses, and offspring.

HISTORY OF INTRAUTERINE NEUROSURGERY IN MAMMALS

Even a cursory glance at most neuroembryological textbooks reveals that knowledge of the basic principles of neurogenesis has been based primarily on experimental studies of amphibian and avian embryos [2,3,4]. Most of this information was obtained either by direct observation of developing embryos or by surgical manipulations of developmental processes that were considered impossible or impractical in mammalian embryos. However, it was suspected from the start that the mammalian brain may develop according to some additional rules, different sequences of developmental events, and slower tempo of maturity so that numerous attempts have been made to find a way to surgically manipulate mammalian embryos. For example, some initial efforts were directed towards producing extrauterine pregnancies with the idea that an embryo in the abdominal cavity would allow more convenient visualization or better access to the fetus. Other attempts at prenatal surgery were restricted to relatively simple procedures, for example, amputation of limbs or extirpation of gonads [5]. No microsurgery was employed and the neurosurgical procedures themselves were rather crude, for example, transection of the spinal cord [6,7]. In the fifties, Hess began a series of eye enucleations in guinea pig embryos to study the effect on visual centers in the brain. In general, lesions of the fetal brain were performed on small rodents. The procedure and approach required little care for the uterus and failures were simply not recorded [8]. More recently, the procedures for neural lesions in the rodent fetal brain have been refined and success in terms of obtaining new neurobiological data has improved [9]. However, the scope, procedures, anesthesia, techniques, and management used in small rodents remain totally different from the problems encountered in performance of neurosurgery in large primates.

More complex neurosurgery on large mammals was initiated in the forties by Donald Barron at Yale University Medical School. He and his colleagues in the Department of Anatomy performed operations that involved craniotomies and resections and/or undercutting of the cerebral neocortex in fetal sheep in the second half of gestation [10,11]. However, most of these early studies unfortunately did not provide details on technical procedures or systematic analysis of the success of surgery on either fetus or mother. The experimental design of these and other studies was such that they did not expect to produce postnatal survival of the operated fetuses. Rather they were intended for acute physiological studies and direct observations of the effect of the lesion during a relatively short period following surgery. These studies also did not furnish neurobiological data of significance comparable to findings from experimental manipulations on avian and amphibian embryos. The field was simply not ready for this type of research in mammals. The need, however, was there.

The modern era of fetal surgery, which permits complex operations *in utero* on larger mammals with a reasonable survival rate, started in the sixties. These were performed on dogs, sheep, and more recently monkeys, cats and rabbits. In primates, a wide variety of surgical procedures was carried out ranging from compression of the umbilical cord [12,13,14] to removal of various organs [15]. Thymectomy was perhaps the most traumatic of surgical procedures performed on primate fetuses, involving, as it does, a tracheotomy and lengthy periods outside the uterus [16]. Other procedures included adrenalectomy [17], fetal radiography [18], and bilateral occlusion of the carotid arteries and jugular veins [12,20].

SURGICAL TECHNIQUES FOR FETAL NEUROSURGERY
IN RHESUS MONKEY

In spite of the variety of surgical procedures carried out on primate fetuses, neurosurgery was not attempted until the mid-seventies. The first report of neurosurgical intervention is that of Taub et al., [21] describing his initial efforts to perfom dorsal rhizotomies and Goldman's early prefrontal surgeries. No single methodological breakthrough was responsible for the introduction of prenatal neurosurgery in primates. At the beginning, we adopted many maneuvers and small but important improvements mentioned to us generously by our colleague, Dr. R. Myers, who had performed several types of surgery on rhesus monkey fetuses or their blood supply *in utero*. We also benefited from personal communication with Dr. B. Jackson (Dept. of Surgery, Brown University, Providence, R.I.) and P. Saghal (New England Research Primate Center, Southborough, Mass.) and Dr. J. Bacher (Division of Research Resources, Bethesda, Md.), regarding procedures for cesarean section.

The main improvements responsible for the success of fetal surgery were the use of intratracheal halothane–oxygen anesthesia, which permits good oxygenation of both mother and fetus during prolonged surgeries, rigorous enforcement of sterile procedure, careful selection of incision, preservation of amniotic fluid, appropriate and careful suturing of fetal membranes, and finally the use of systemically and locally applied muscle relaxants before, during, and after surgery, to prevent abortion. Progress in experimental prenatal surgery was basically limited by problems in handling the uterus, fetal circulation, and, in particular, placental attachments rather than by problems in fetal surgery itself. The fast growing epithelium of the skin and other fetal tissues bathed in the sterile amniotic fluid provided nearly ideal conditions for surgery and fast healing [21]. Furthermore, incisions in the uterine wall heal fast and extremely well in pregnant primates [22].

Our usual procedure is as follows. Pregnancy in rhesus monkey lasts 165 days. So far, for practical reasons as well as to suit our research goals, most of our surgeries have been carried out between embryonic (E) day E90 and E120. The youngest fetus operated on was E60 and the oldest, E152. Pregnant rhesus monkeys of specified gestational ages are prepared for uterine surgery by an intramuscular injection of the smooth muscle relaxant, Vasodilan (isoxusprine HCl 10 mg/day), sedated with ketamine (3 mg/kg body wt), and anesthetized by a halothane–oxygen mixture administered intratracheally.

Physiological saline and dextrose is routinely administered intravenously. The abdomen is dressed in preparation for cesarean section. The abdominal wall is cut sagittally to expose the uterus. The uterus is lifted from the abdominal cavity. This is important particularly at later stages of pregnancy when it should be padded with gauze soaked in warm sterile saline solution. The exposed uterine surface is sprayed with Cyclane (Merck, Sharpe and Dohme) to diminish contraction and the incision site is determined by gentle palpation in order to locate the edges of the placentas. This procedure requires particular attention since the rhesus monkey usually has two placental lobes that can vary in shape and size. The palpation of the uterus is most critical for the success of the surgery, and only judgment backed by experience and considerable trial and error has been responsible for our current good results. Initially, we lost fetuses following surgery if the incision was too close to the placenta or if the blade or any instrument touched its edge. Frequently during exploratory palpation, the uterine contractions may obscure the exact location of placental borders. In such cases, one should wait several minutes until contractions subside and try again until localization is reasonably sure.

Once the line of the incision is determined, it is marked by placing temporary sutures at each end of the prospective cut. The size of incision, of course, depends on the stage of pregnancy but a general rule of thumb is a length of about 30% more than the diameter of the fetal skull to allow for subsequent replacement if contractions of the uterine wall develop. After a small exploratory incision is made to expose the fetal membranes, which are transparent, a small hole is made, a catheter is placed into the amniotic cavity, and amniotic fluid is removed and stored in sterile syringes. Depending upon the size of the uterus, we remove between 10 and 75 ml of fluid. After that, the uterine incision is enlarged by simultaneously cutting the uterine wall and fetal membranes in one or both directions using scissors under direct visual guidance to assure that no placental tissue is damaged. Following the cut, the fetal membranes and the uterine wall are sutured together by performing a continuous stitch with No. 000 gut to form a buttonhole-like opening (Figure 1). This latter step is made in an attempt to diminish the possibility of subsequent abortion that may be caused by separation of the fetal membranes and detachment of placenta from the uterine wall, as well as to prevent bleeding from damaged uterine blood vessels [23].

The buttonhole-like suture makes replacement of the fetus and subsequent closure of the uterine wall easier and cleaner. The

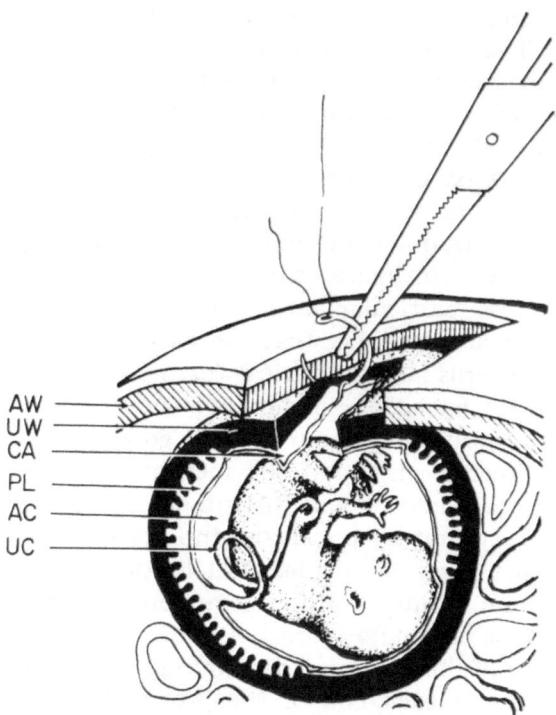

AW
UW
CA
PL
AC
UC

Figure 1. A schematic drawing of the monkey fetus in the uterine cavity in the midgestational period. The incision on the uterus is placed between the two placental lobes and running stitches are carried along the edges of the cut to attach the uterine wall (UW) and chorioallantoic membranes (CA). The sutured buttonhole-like opening prevents detachment of the placenta from the uterine wall and subsequent bleeding from the uterine wall which, before this procedure was introduced, had been the main cause of abortion following prenatal surgery. Furthermore, lifting of the sutured hole (as illustrated in Figure 2) helps to preserve amniotic fluid, which is important for survival of the fetus. Abbreviations: AC, amniotic cavity; AW, abdominal wall; PL, placenta; UC, umbilical cord.

level of the incision can be elevated by lifting two temporary silk sutures placed at edges of the cut (Figure 2). This maneuver may also save some fluid, but it is adequate only for simple experiments such as injection of substances into the eye or eye enucleation. For more complex neurosurgical procedures, such as extensive ablation of the cerebral cortex or insertion of a micropipette into the brain for the purpose of injecting various substances, the fetus may be removed fully from the uterus and placed on a stable platform fixed to the surgical table with a flexibar and covered with sterile gauze soaked

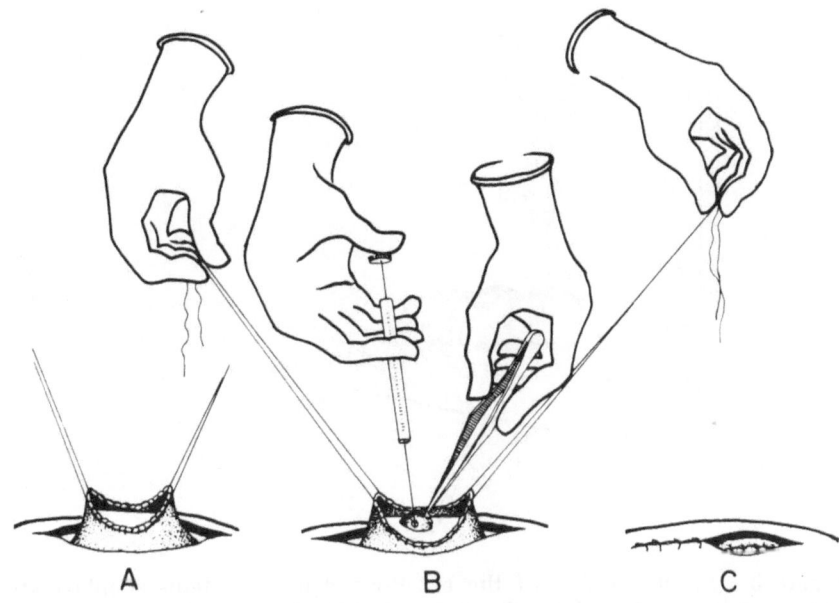

Figure 2.   This diagram illustrates the simplest procedure which we have used to inject one eye of the fetus whose body essentially remains in the uterine cavity. The buttonhole-like opening is lifted by two silk threads to preserve amniotic fluid. This initial procedure has now been modified to allow removal of the fetus from the uterus which permits more complex prenatal neurosurgery.

with warm physiological saline (eg, Figure 3). The blood supply during fetal surgery is preserved via the umbilical cord. We are able to perform several types of extensive surgical procedures on the marsupialized or exteriorized monkey fetus—including eye injections with radioactive tracers, enucleation of one or both eyes, injection and resections of large and/or whole prefrontal, motor, sensory, parietal, and visual cortical areas in one and/or both cerebral hemispheres. For injections into various cerebral structures, a carrier from a stereotaxic apparatus is fixed to the surgical table and fitted with a micromanipulator enabling the placement of a micropipette or microsyringe into the desired target (Figure 3).

   For resection of large areas of cortex, the dural membrane is incised and flapped. The cortical surface in the fetus is covered by a highly vascular pial membrane that gives the brain a very different and more bloody appearance than in the mature brain. Although bleeding can be greater than in neonates or adults, it is also easily

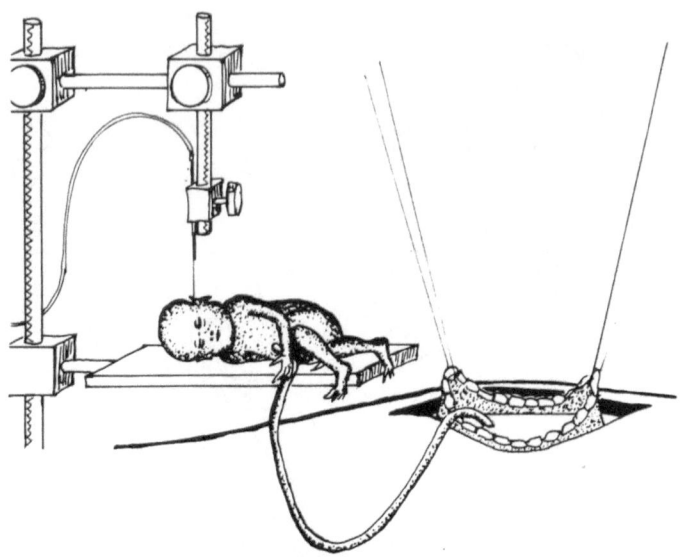

Figure 3. An illustration of the exteriorized monkey fetus at midgestation, placed on the fixed platform. The removal of the fetus avoids movements caused by the mother's breathing. This is helpful for precise localization of intra-cerebral injections. The fetus, hydrated by constant moistening with warm (36°C) saline solution, can be kept outside of the uterus for about one hour in order to perform complex surgical procedures such as partial eye enucleation, resection of the various cortical fields, or slow injection into the inner ear as illustrated in this drawing.

controlled by electrocautery. For most of gestation and until the end of the second trimester, the cortical surface is basically lissencephalic, that is, without the deep sulci and gyri that form cytoarchitectonic boundaries in the adult brain. However from about E90 on, the brain has already formed its major lobes and small "dimples" begin to denote the location where landmark sulci will form, thus making it possible to remove territories that are anlagen for specific cortical fields in adults. The still rather gelatinous fetal cortex is removed by aspiration with a liberal use of electrocauterization or pressure to prevent bleeding. Following resection, the meningeal membranes, subcutaneous tissue, and scalp are sutured in layers with No. 0000 or No. 000 gut, respectively. In some experiments, the fetus was outside the uterus for between 40 to 90 minutes at room temperature while neurosurgery was performed and then returned to the uterus with no apparent ill effect [24-29].

After neurosurgery or injection of isotopes and enzymes, fetuses are replaced into the uterine cavity and fetal membranes and the uterine wall are sutured with two layers of stitches. Before completely closing the wound, amniotic fluid is injected back into the uterus and then the last stitches are taken. Peritoneal membranes, abdominal muscles, and skin are sutured in a manner routine for cesarean sections. Postoperatively, mothers are injected daily with 10 mg (I.M.) of Vasodilan to abolish posttraumatic uterine contractions and to prevent abortion. The survival of the fetus can be monitored by stethoscope and its growth checked by x-ray and ultrasound.

Fetuses are delivered by a second cesarean section at various intervals following surgery dictated by the design of our experiments. Even when we plan postnatal survival of the offspring, cesarean section is usually performed one to two weeks before term to avoid unplanned damage to the operated fetus by the harshness of a spontaneous delivery. To prevent possible damage of the offspring by the mother, particularly in cases of larger cortical lesions, the newborns are separated from the mother on the first day and bottle fed. With appropriate care, fetuses delivered up to 2.5 weeks before term can survive and develop to infancy or maturity. Larger bone defects on the skull do not close up, but dura mater and the scalp heal better than in similar procedures performed postnatally. There is usually little effect on the baby's progress and gain in weight, compared with normal offspring. The behavior of newborns that were operated on *in utero* is of course carefully monitored after delivery.

SUCCESS RATE AND PROSPECTS FOR PRENATAL NEUROSURGERY IN THE FIELD OF DEVELOPMENTAL NEUROBIOLOGY

Fetal neurosurgeries in our research program have an average 65 to 70% overall success in more than 100 procedures. The survival, however, varies considerably according to the type of neurosurgery performed and stage of pregnancy. For example, eye injection which requires one-day survival has a 90 to 95% rate of success, eye enucleation at the midgestational period has about a 75 to 80% rate of success, whereas fetuses with bilateral cortical removal during the first half of gestation have about a 60% chance of survival. Fortunately, in our experiments even unsuccessful surgeries, which result in abortion, usually provide fetal brains that can be used for various normative studies such as routine histology, Golgi impregnation, or histochemical and biochemical analysis of brain tissue. We have not lost a single mother due to surgical intervention on the fetus and some have had up to five consecutive pregnancies.

It should be emphasized that prenatal surgery in our laboratories is carried out in order to study mechanisms of formation of neuronal connections or with the intention of manipulating normal developmental processes as a way of gaining insight into developmental mechanisms and functional consequences of fetal brain injuries. Our experiments have not been designed to learn about or improve methods of corrective neurosurgery. Nevertheless, our experience clearly demonstrates that it is feasible to perform relatively complex and prolonged neurosurgical procedures on the brains of non-human primates with a rather small risk to the mother and perhaps an acceptable risk to the fetus.

The causes of fetal death in our series cannot presently be determined with any degree of security since the experimental design did not allow appropriate testing of the procedure or the optimal conditions for pathological examination. We also did not perform sham operations as they would be too costly and time consuming. However, we learned that the first three days after surgery and the week around term are critical periods. In some cases of cortical ablation, fetal death may occur due to secondary damage to the brain, such as intracranial hemorrhage or injury to brainstem vital centers as a result of inadvertent twisting of the neck during surgery or during replacement of the fetus into the uterus. As our considerable numbers of surviving fetuses attest, cortical removal alone is not life-threatening. The most likely cause of death in some, if not most of our cases, may be damage to the maternal environment, for example, disruption in placental perfusion, loss of amniotic fluid, detachment and/or bleeding of the placenta, and, in particular, irritability and contraction of the uterine muscles which could compress and asphyxiate the developing fetus. However, until these various causes and variables are analyzed more systematically and with adequate controls, it is not possible to specify with any level of confidence the main reasons for abortions in our experiments.

In spite of a 25 to 30% overall mortality rate, prenatal neurosurgery has become an indispensible tool for the study of brain development in non-human primates [24,25,27-29,30-32]. Essentially similar procedures have been used in pregnant rabbits [33] and cats [34,35] although the double hornshape of the uterus and multiple fetuses in these species obviously require appropriate modifications. The procedures presently available allow performance of at least two types of studies: (1) acute, short-range experiments such as electrophysiological recordings, use of anterograde and retrograde axonal transport methods for tracing neuronal connections; and (2) long-term survival experiments for the analysis of structural and functional consequences of selective and well defined prenatal brain lesions. Both types of experiments have already furnished neurobiological data that were not possible or even suspected just a few years ago.

SELECTED NEUROBIOLOGICAL FINDINGS
AND PROSPECTS FOR RESEARCH
USING PRENATAL NEUROSURGERY

Among the findings obtained from fetal surgery that influenced our thinking about normal and pathological development of the primate brain, we shall mention only a few since it is not our intention to review this exciting and fast growing field of neurobiology. The accessibility of the brain opens new possibilities for the study of the timing, sequence, mechanisms, and modifiability of development of cerebral systems that are established in primates before birth.

Perhaps it is worth stating that injections of radioactive tracers into the fetal eye revealed that binocular projections from the eyes initially overlap before they segregate into appropriate territories in the lateral geniculate nucleus and ocular dominance columns in the visual cortex [30,36]. This provided the first evidence that synaptogenesis in the primate visual system proceeds in two phases, a finding which has considerable theoretical significance. The first tracing studies of frontal cortical connections in fetal primates showed that the adult columnar pattern of callosal axons [26] and the fenestrated pattern of the adult corticostriatal axons [37] are achieved at least two months before birth. These results could not be discovered in primates without the use of intrauterine surgery. We have also shown that enucleation of one eye before birth permanently changes the adult cellular organization of synaptic connectivity of the visual cortex [27,28]. The most notable alterations are that (1) the lateral geniculate nucleus develops only two cellular layers and one intralaminar fiber band instead of the normal six layers and five interlaminar bands, (2) the optic tract of the remaining eye contains supernumerary axons, (3) aberrant synaptic connections are formed between the intact eye and geniculate neurons that have not been deprived of their normal input, and (4) ocular dominance columns fail to develop in the visual cortex.

The use of prenatal resection of the cerebral cortex with subsequent survival of the offspring revealed a considerable capacity of developing corticocortical and corticostriatal connections for modifiability and changes in the pattern of their terminal fields [31]. Thus, when the dorsolateral prefrontal cortex in one cerebral hemisphere is removed six weeks before birth and the fetus survives to postnatal ages, neurons of the corresponding cortex in the intact hemisphere issue a greatly expanded projection to the contralateral caudate nucleus in addition to the normal projection to the ipsilateral neostriatum [24]. Likewise, callosal fibers find their way to regions of the cortex where they normally do not project [37]. These studies provide direct evidence for lesion-induced neuronal rearrangement in the primate telencephalon. Finally, it should be mentioned that monkeys which have sustained prenatal injuries of the frontal cortex show remarkable sparing of delayed response capacity compared to animals sustaining brain damage of the very same region as young adults. The implications of these findings for neonatal neurology and neuropathology are obvious [38]. We can expect that our knowledge of pathogenesis of neonatal lesions and interpretation of neuropathological findings will be enhanced by experimental work on fetal monkeys at precisely defined critical periods.

Fetal neurosurgery has already yielded important basic developmental information, as well as provided a critical link between experimental studies on the non-mammalian brain and those obtained from human postmortem material. Theoretically, one can expect to perform transplantations of the kind accomplished in avian brain [39] or implantation of various devices for monitoring cerebral blood flow or chemical composition of cerebrospinal fluid. However, at present, the type of surgical manipulations that can be performed in amphibian and avian experimental neuroembryology is still much more complex than those so far performed in any mammals; yet, apart from technical difficulties that are eminently solvable, the approach is strategically the same. However, the type of neurobiological data that is obtained is frequently different since the mammalian brain and, in particular, the primate brain develops and reacts to injury in a unique way. Thus, species can now be evaluated and taken into consideration in understanding pathogenesis of perinatal injuries to the human brain in a way that was not possible before.

REFERENCES

1. Harrison, M. The fetus becomes patient. Phi Delta Epsilon Lecture, University of California, San Francisco, 1983.
2. Detwiler, S. R. *Neuroembryology. An Experimental Study.* New York: MacMillan Publishing Co. 1936.
3. Harrison, R. G. On the origin and development of the nervous system studied by the methods of experimental embryology. *Proc. Roy. Soc. (London) Sec. B. 118:*155-196, 1935.
4. Jacobson, M. *Development Neurobiology*, New York: Plenum Press, 1978.
5. Hess, A. The experimental embryology of the foetal nervous system. *Biol. Rev. 32:*231-260, 1957.
6. Hooker, D., and Nicholas, J. S. Spinal cord section in rat fetuses. *J. Comp. Neurol. 50:*413-467, 1930.
7. Gerard, R. W., and Grinker, R. P. Regenerative possibilities of the central system. *Arch Neurol. Psychiat. 26:*469-484, 1931.
8. DeMayer, W., and Baird, I. Techinique of prenatal neurosurgical observation on rat fetuses and obtaining postnatal survival. *Teratology 7:*89-98, 1973.
9. Miller, B. F., and Lund, R. D. The pattern of retinotectal connections in albino rats can be modified by fetal surgery. *Brain Res, 91:*119-125, 1975.
10. Barcroft, J., and Barron, D. H. Observation on the functional development of the foetal brain. *J. Comp. Neurol. 77:*431-454, 1942.
11. Barron, D. H. An experimental analysis of some factors involved in the development of the fissure patterns of cerebral cortex. *J. Exp. Zool. 113:*553-581, 1950.
12. Myers, R. E. Brain pathology following fetal vascular occlusion: An experimental study. *Invest. Ophthal. 8:*41-50, 1969.
13. Myers, R. E. Brain damage induced by umbilical cord compression at different gestational ages in monkeys. *Second Conf. Exper. Med.,* 1971.
14. Myers, R. E. Two patterns of perinatal brain damage and their conditions of occurrence. *Amer J. Ob. Gyn. 112:*246-276, 1972.
15. Chez, R. A., and Hutchinson, D. L. The use of experimental surgical techniques in the pregnant *Macaca mulatta. Ann. N.Y. Acad. Sci.* 249-253, 1969.
16. Hess, A. Optic centers and pathways after eye removal in fetal guinea pigs. *J. Comp. Neuro. 109:*91-115, 1958.
17. Marshall C. J., Jr., and Silverstein, A. M. Surgical approaches to the study of fetal immunology in primate animals. *Ann. N.Y. Acad. Sci. 162:*254-266, 1969.
18. Mueller-Heuback, E., Myers, R. E., and Adamsons, K. Effects of adrenalectomy on pregnancy length in the rhesus monkey. *Amer. J. Ob. Gyn. 112:*221-226, 1972.
19. Michejda, M., Bacher, J., and Johnson, D. Surgical approaches in fetal radiography and the study of skeletal age in *Macaca mulatta. J. Med. Primatology 9:*50-61, 1980.
20. Myers, R. E. Fetal asphyxia and perinatal brain damage. In *Perinatal Factors Affecting Human Development.* PAHO Scientific Publ. No. 185:205-214, 1969.
21. Somasundaram, K., and Prathap, K. Intra-uterine healing of skin wounds in rabbit fetuses. *J. Path. 100:*81-86, 1969.

22. Hartman, C. G. Regeneration of the monkey uterus after surgical removal of the endometrium and accidental endometriosis. *West. J. Surg. Obstet. Gynecol. 52*:87–102, 1944.

23. Jackson, B. T., and Egdahl. The performance of complex foetal operations *in utero* without amniotic fluid loss or other disturbances of foetal-maternal relationships. *Surgery 48*:564–570, 1960.

24. Goldman, P. S. Neuronal plasticity in primate telencephalon: anomalous crossed cortico-caudate projections induced by prenatal removal of frontal association cortex. *Science 202*:768–776, 1978.

25. Goldman, P. S., and Galkin, T. W. Prenatal removal of frontal association cortex in the rhesus monkey: anatomical and functional consequences in postnatal life. *Brain Res. 52*:451–485, 1978.

26. Goldman-Rakic, P. S. Prenatal formation of cortical input and development of cytoarchitectonic compartments in the neostriatum of rhesus monkey. *J. Neurosci. 1*:721–735, 1981.

27. Rakic, P. Development of visual centers in the primate brain depends on binocular competition before birth. *Science 214*:928–931, 1981.

28. Rakic, P., and Riley, K. P. Regulation of axon number in primate optic nerve by binocular competition. *Nature* (London) *305*:135–137, 1983.

29. Shatz, C., and Rakic, P. The genesis of efferent connections from the visual cortex of the fetal monkey. *J. Comp. Neurol. 196*:287–307, 1981.

30. Rakic, P. Prenatal genesis of connections subserving ocular dominance in the rhesus monkey. *Nature 261*:467–471, 1976.

31. Rakic, P., and Goldman-Rakic, P. S. Development and modifiability of the cerebral cortex. *Neurosc. Res. Program Bull. 20*:429–611, 1982.

32. Taub, E., Barro, G., Miller, E., Perrella, P. N., Jakniunas, A., Goldman, P. S., Petras, J. M., Darrow, C. C., and Martin, D. F. Feasibility of spinal cord or brain surgery in fetal rhesus monkeys. Soc. Neurosci., Fourth Ann. Meet., 1974.

33. Distel, H., and Hollander, H. Autoradiographic tracing of developing subcortical projections of the occipital region in fetal rabbits. *J. Comp. Neurol. 192*:505–518, 1980.

34. Shatz, C. Prenatal development of the cat's retinogeniculate pathway. *J. Neurosci. 3*:482–499, 1983.

35. Williams, R. W., Bastiani, M. J., and Chalupa, L. M. Loss of axons in cat optic nerve following fetal unilateral enucleation: An electromicroscopic analysis. *J. Neurosci. 3*:133–144, 1983.

36. Rakic, P. Prenatal development of the visual system in the rhesus monkey. *Phil. Trans. Roy. Soc. Lond. Sec. B 278*:245–260, 1977.

37. Goldman-Rakic, P. S. Development and plasticity of primate frontal association cortex. In: *The Organization of the Cerebral Cortex*, edited by F. O. Schmitt. Cambridge, Mass.: MIT Press, 1981.

38. Volpe, J. J. *Neurology of the Newborn.* Philadelphia: W. B. Saunders Co., 1981.

39. LeDouarin, N. M. The ontogeny of the neural crest in avian chimaeras. *Nature* (London) *286*:633–669, 1980.

40. Kraner, K. L. Intrauterine fetal surgery. *Adv. Vet. Sci. 10*:1–22, 1965.

41. Morishima, H. O., Hyman, A. I., Adamson, K. Jr., and James, L. S. Anesthetic management for fetal operation in the subhuman primate. *Amer. J. Ob. Gyn. 112*:221–226, 1971.

42. Nicholas, J. S. Notes on the application of experimental methods upon mammalian embryos. *Anat. Rec. 31*:385-394, 1925.
43. Nicholas, J. S. Experimental approaches to problems of early development in the rat. *Quart. Rev. Biol. 22*:179-195, 1947.
44. Rakic, P. Genesis of visual connections in the rhesus monkey. In: *Developmental Biology of Visual System*, edited by R. Freeman. New York: Plenum Press, 1979.
45. Sopher, D. A study of wound healing in the foetal tissues of the cynomolgus monkey. In: *Breeding Simians for Developmental Biology. Laboratory Animal Handbooks 6*:327-335, 1975.

CHAPTER 2

Pathogenesis of Perinatal Hypoxic–Ischemic Brain Damage

Robert C. Vannucci, M.D.

INTRODUCTION

The brain damage which results from a combination of systemic hypoxia and reduced cerebral blood flow (ischemia) in the fetus and newborn infant remains a major cause of chronic neurological disability. *Hypoxia* denotes a partial lack of oxygen with or without concurrent accumulation of carbon dioxide. *Asphyxia* is that state in which pulmonary or placental gas exchange ceases, resulting in progressive hypoxemia or anoxemia combined with hypercapnia. *Ischemia* is a reduction in or cessation of blood flow. It rarely occurs during the perinatal period without antecedent hypoxia or asphyxia.

NEUROPATHOLOGY OF HUMAN PERINATAL CEREBRAL HYPOXIA-ISCHEMIA

Perinatal hypoxic-ischemic brain damage and the associated neurological entities of cerebral palsy, epilepsy, and mental retardation has been known since Little's classic treatise on the subject in 1861 [1]. Since then, numerous investigators have confirmed Little's findings and have expanded our knowledge on the early and late pathological reactions of the brain to perinatal hypoxic-ischemic stress [2-5]. In the past, the neuropathological endstage of perinatal

Perinatal Neurology and Neurosurgery. Edited by R. A. Thompson, J. R. Green, and S. D. Johnsen. Copyright © 1985 by Spectrum Publications, Inc.

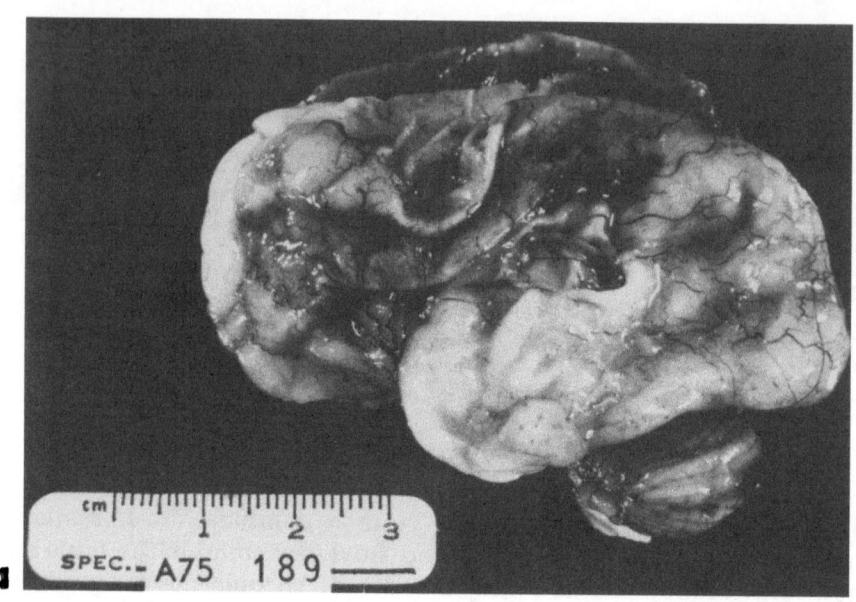

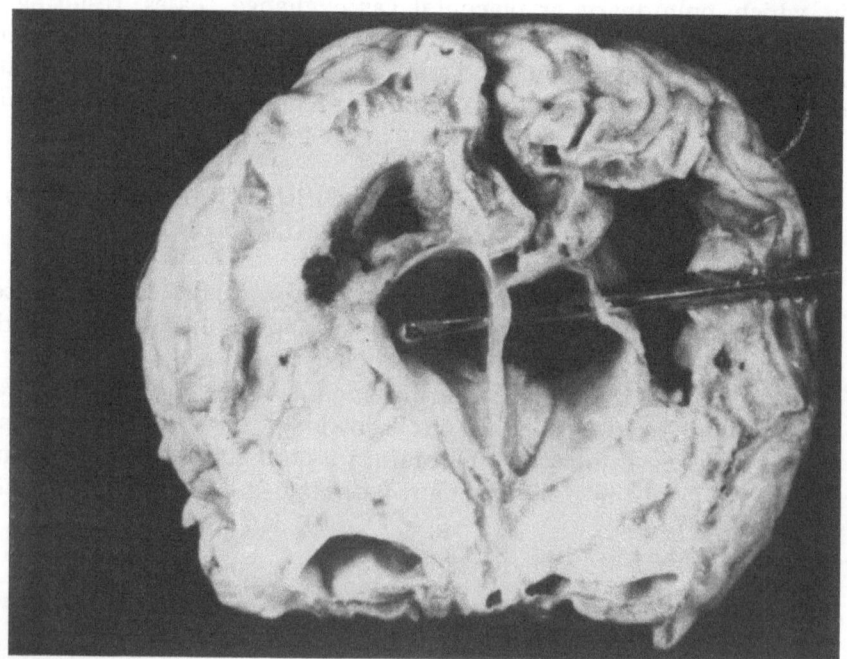

brain damage has been inferred primarily from circumstantial evidence [6]. Despite such difficulty, one now can identify several specific long-standing morphological abnormalities consistently implying that they have resulted from early hypoxic-ischemic injury. Such lesions include selective neuronal necrosis and/or infarction with secondary atrophy of the cerebral cortex (ulegyria), subcortical and periventricular necrosis with secondary sclerosis and cyst formation (leukomalacia and porencephaly), and necrosis with secondary degeneration of the basal ganglia and thalamus, brainstem or cerebellum (Figures 1 and 2). These pathological entities are manifested by specific functional alterations in motor control and cognition during life [7].

The neuropathological lesions resulting from perinatal cerebral hypoxia-ischemia largely occur in a vascular distribution. In addition, the locations of the lesions are dependent upon the gestational age of the infant at the time of the insult. In infants whose gestational ages are 36 weeks or greater at the time of hypoxia-ischemia, infarction occurs which often is confined to the cerebral cortex and to the adjacent subcortical white matter. In infants whose gestational ages are less than 36 weeks at the time of the insult, infarction occurs in the deep (periventricular) white matter structures. Both the cerebral, cortical, and white matter lesions are situated within arterial boundary zones—areas which are the most distant from the origin of their blood supply and, therefore, are most vulnerable to ischemia [8,9]. As in the adult, the arterial boundary zones in the term infant are located between the three major cerebral arteries (anterior, middle, and posterior) with secondary boundary zones at the depth of cortical sulci [10]. In premature infants, the most prominent arterial boundary zones exist in the periventricular white matter adjacent to the external angles of the lateral ventricles (Figure 3) [2]. These zones are situated 3 to 10 mm from the ventricular wall and lie between the terminal distributions of ventriculofugal arteries

Figure 1.   (a) Gross brain specimen showing ulgyria. Shown is the brain of a premature infant which demonstrates gross distortion of gyri and sulci primarily in the distribution of the middle cerebral artery of the left cerebral hemisphere. Microscopic examination revealed abnormalities characteristic of ulegyria. (b) Gross brain specimen showing ulegyria. Shown is the brain of an infant who expired at three years of age and who previously had sustained both perinatal asphyxia and intraventricular hemorrhage. Note the cerebral cortical and subcortical atrophy associated with lateral ventricular enlargement. The porencephalic cyst on the right communicates with the ipsilaterial lateral ventricle (rod).

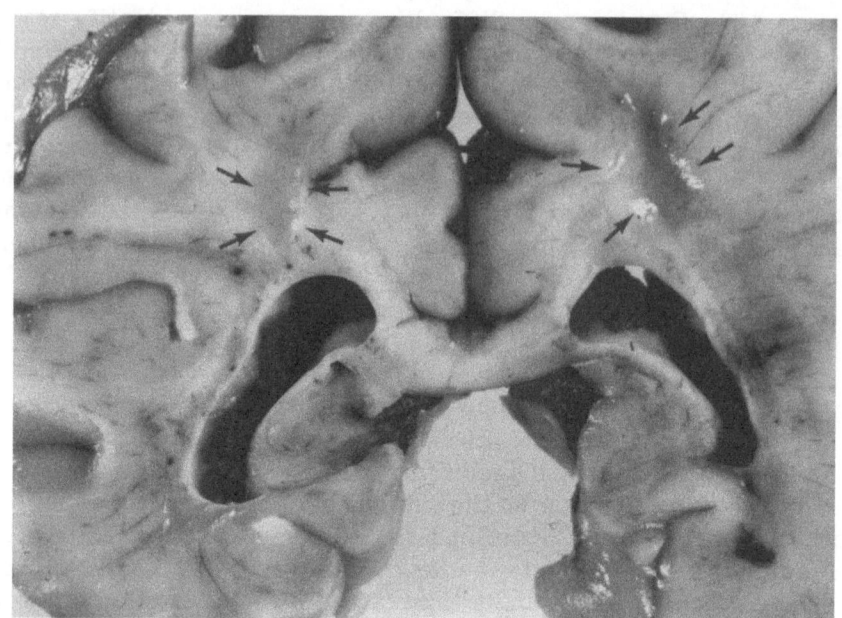

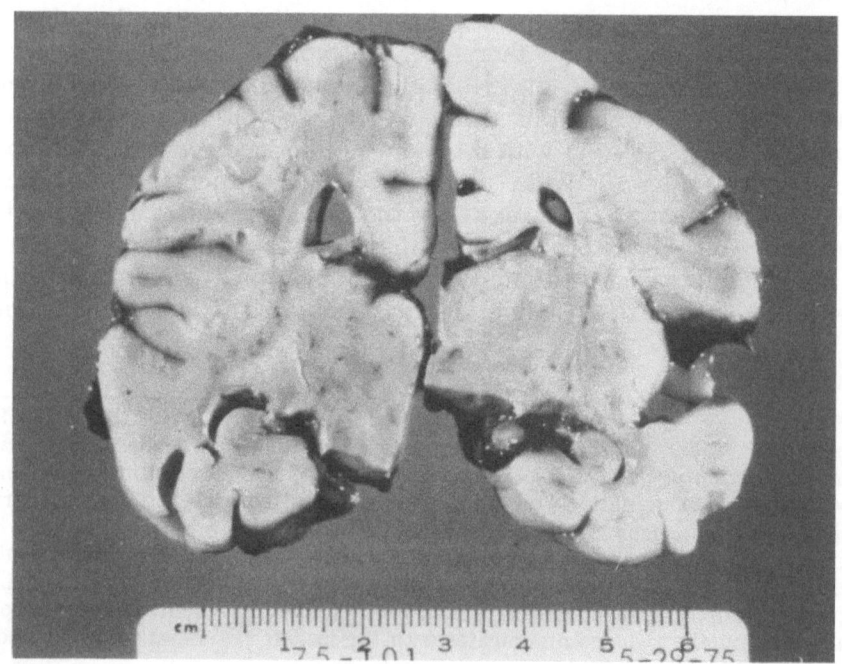

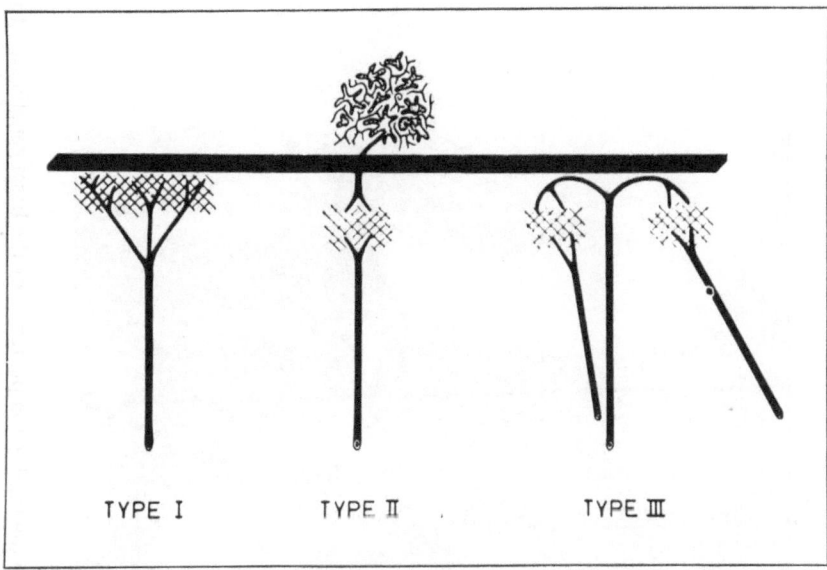

TYPE I   TYPE II   TYPE III

Figure 3. Diagram of periventricular arterial boundary zones. Type I, at the ventricular wall itself; Type II, between deeply penetrating (ventriculopedal) medullary artery and ventriculofugal branch from a choroid plexus artery; Type III, between ventriculofugal and ventriculopedal end-branches of deeply penetrating arteries. From DeReuck et al. [12] with permission.

which course from the choroid plexus peripherally to meet penetrating branches of long parenchymal (ventriculopedal) arteries originating at the surface of the cerebral cortex [11-13]. The ventriculofugal vessels increase in number with increasing gestational age; therefore, their relative paucity in the premature infant targets the periventricular white matter as a structure prone to ischemic infarction [10]. Sparing of the cerebral cortex from hypoxic-ischemic damage in the premature infant may relate to the presence

Figure 2. (a) Brain specimen showing periventricular leukomalacia. Shown is a posterior coronal section of the brain of a premature infant which demonstrates softening of the white matter (arrows) within both cerebral hemispheres. The lateral ventricles are mildly dilated. (b) Brain specimen showing periventricular leukomalacia. Shown is an anterior coronal section of the brain of an infant who was born prematurely and who sustained episodes of apnea, bradycardia, and hypotension. The specimen shows bilateral white matter cavitation.

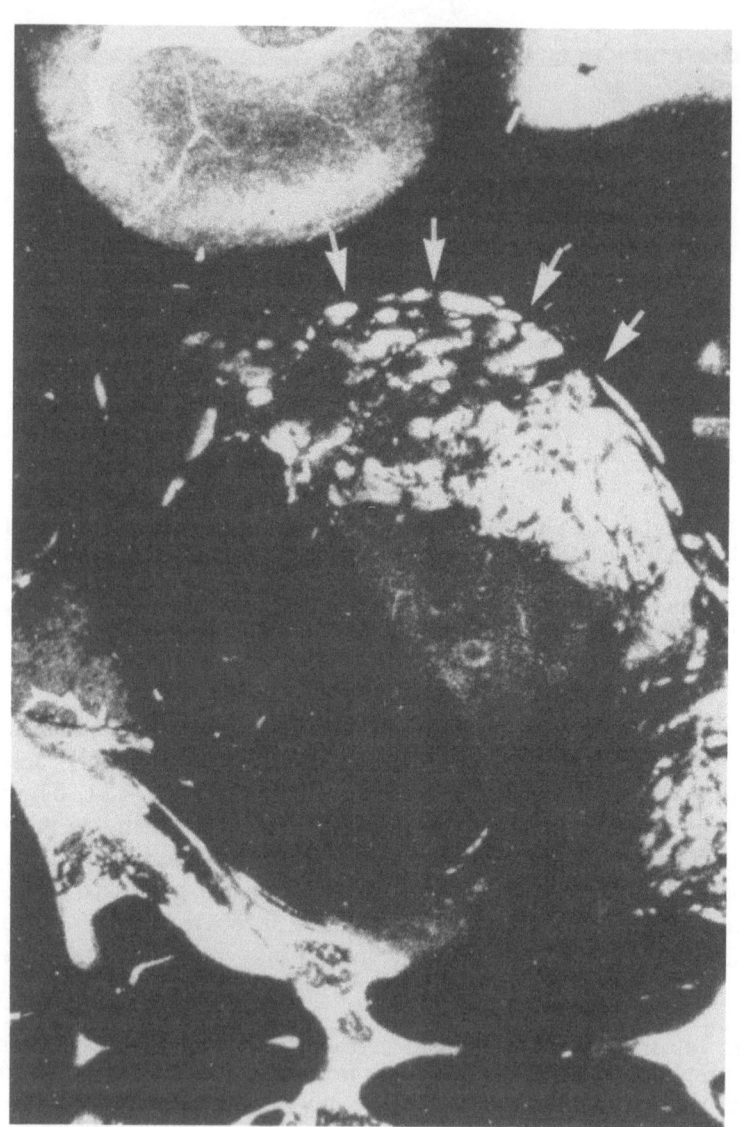

Figure 4. Coronal section of brain showing status marmoratus. Note the marbled appearance of the basal ganglia structures, especially the putamen (arrows).

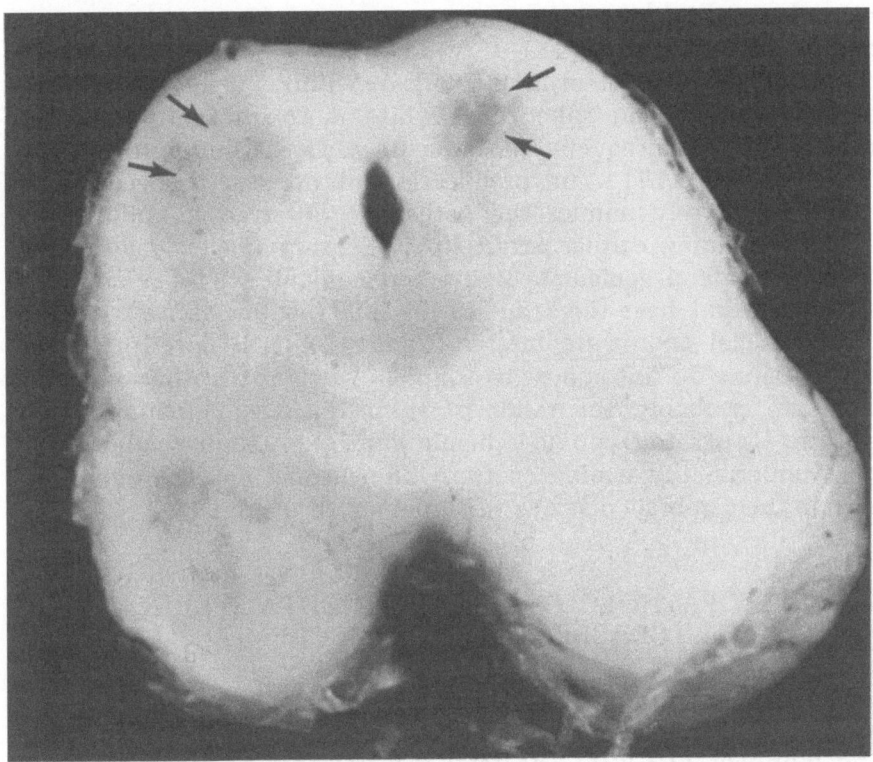

Figure 5. Coronal section of the brainstem showing hypoxic-ischemic brain damage. The infant died acutely at four months of age after cardiopulmonary arrest complicating acute laryngotracheobronchitis. Note discoloration and necrosis of the inferior colliculi (arrows). From Leech and Alvord [16], with permission.

of a rich vascular anastomosis between arteries supplying the meninges and the anterior, middle, and posterior cerebral arteries. These anastomoses are prominent in the immature brain but essentially disappear by term.

Status marmoratus of the basal ganglia and thalamus is a characteristic, albeit uncommon, neuropathological manifestation of perinatal hypoxia-ischemia. Grossly, the basal ganglia and thalamus exhibit patchy marbled appearance, which histologically is identified as areas of hypermyelination (Figure 4). Under the electron microscope, these hypermyelinated areas are actually myelinated astrocytic processes rather than neurons [14]. The lesions typically result from an asphyxial insult occurring in term infants but also have been described in infants in whom insults occurred as late as three months following birth [15].

Prominent brainstem injury with or without involvement of the cerebral cortex and subcortical white matter recently has been reported as a consequence of an acute asphyxial insult to the new-born brain [16,17]. The predilection of damage to occur in the brainstem closely mimics the pathology observed in children and adults sustaining cardiac arrest [18]. Sensory nuclei including the thalamus, lateral geniculate body, and colliculi are those brainstem structures that bear the brunt of the injury with relative sparing of motor nuclei and white matter (Figure 5). It is noteworthy that these lesions do not appear to follow a vascular distribution; rather they are probably the result of an intrinsic vulnerability of the specific tissues to hypoxic-ischemic damage. A similar vulnerability may underlie the laminar pattern of neuronal necrosis commonly seen in the cerebral cortex as a component of ulegyria.

NEUROPATHOLOGY OF EXPERIMENTAL PERINATAL CEREBRAL HYPOXIA-ISCHEMIA

In experimental animals, structural brain damage from perinatal hypoxia-ischemia has been investigated in rats, guinea pigs, sheep, and monkeys [19-22]. The fetal and newborn rhesus monkey has been studied extensively because of its similarities to man with respect to the physiology of reproduction and to its neuroanatomy at the time of birth. In addition, the animal's size and neurological maturity allow it to be nursed in a manner similar to that of human infants.

Monkey fetuses asphyxiated at birth to the point of apnea and then reanimated by resuscitation exhibit hypotonia, poor coordinated movements, and a loss of postural righting reflexes following the insult [23]. Neuropathological examination at one to three months of age reveals brain damage predominantly in the brainstem and consisting of symmetrical neuronal destruction of the sensory cranial nerve neucle, inferior colliculus, and ventrolateral thalamus (Figure 6). Varying degrees of astrocytosis and vascular proliferation also are seen, depending on how long the animal is asphyxiated. The neuronal lesions do not appear to follow a specific vascular distribution. If severely asphyxiated monkeys are reared for 10 months to 8 years, atrophy of the cerebral hemispheres evolves as the prominent neuropathological feature, with the most severe neuronal

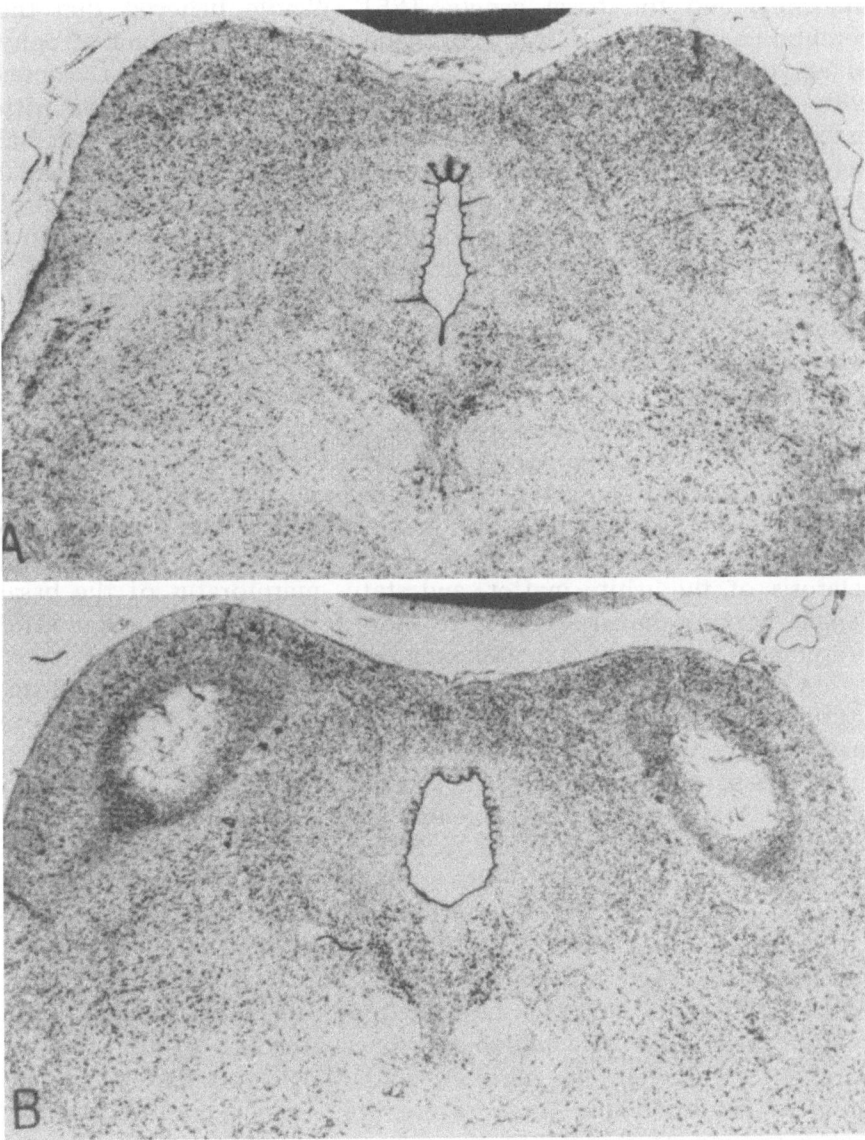

Figure 6. Coronal sections of the brainstem of two monkeys showing hypoxic-ischemic brain damage. Section A is taken at the level of the inferior colliculus of a normal monkey at four years of age. Section B is taken at the same level of a monkey asphyxiated for 14 minutes at birth and sacrificed at the age of four years. Note the bilateral lesions of the central nuclei of the inferior colliculus as represented by cavities. From Windle [24] with permission.

loss in the second and fourth layers of the cerebral cortex, the thalamus, and the basal ganglia [25]. Windle believed that the cerebral cortical damage was a consequence of transneuronal atrophy of nerve fibers that normally connect the brainstem and thalamus with cortical projection areas. Interestingly, such monkeys with extensive postmortem brain damage often appear fairly normal behaviorally. However, detailed examination reveals a lack of manual dexterity and fine motor coordination as well as a reduced level of spontaneous activity, a description that in many ways resembles that applied to children with "attention deficit disorders."

Myers and his colleagues have studied the pattern of brain injury following "prolonged partial asphyxia" [26,27]. Fetal monkeys at term were asphyxiated for 0.5 to 3 hours by constriction of the abdominal aorta above the origins of the uterine vessels. This manipulation led to graded decreases in fetal PA_{O_2} to between 10 and 15 mm Hg and increased in PA_{CO_2} to between 70 and 145 mm Hg. Animals who recovered were reared and later killed, at which time damage was seen mainly in the cerebral hemispheres. The principal lesions consisted of atrophy of the cortical gray matter, sclerosis of the white matter, and status marmoratus of the basal ganglia, lesions almost identical to those found in humans late after presumed perinatal hypoxic-ischemic insults.

In addition, investigators Brann and Myers [28] produced intra-uterine "partial asphyxia" by inducing prolonged (two to four hours) maternal hypotension with halothane. Measurements of fetal oxygen and acid–base balance revealed severe combined (respiratory and metabolic) acidosis and hypoxemia with pH_a below 7.0, PA_{CO_2} above 60 mm Hg and PA_{O_2} below 20 mm Hg in all fetuses. Systemic blood pressure responses to the asphyxial insult were variable but declined to as low as 57% of control. Following delivery and resuscitation, the animals often required prolonged ventilation, developed seizures, and could not be maintained for longer than 96 hours. Neuropathological analysis at that time showed extensive brain swelling and both pale and hemorrhagic necrosis of the cerebral cortices (Figure 7). The monkeys with the lowest systemic blood pressure exhibited the most severe brain damage. Since swelling was a prominent feature of the neuropathology, the investigators speculated that brain edema was a primary event leading, in turn, to impaired cerebral blood flow and secondary cerebral necrosis (see below).

Based on his investigations spanning 15 years, Myers has proposed that the distribution of brain damage seen in the perinatal

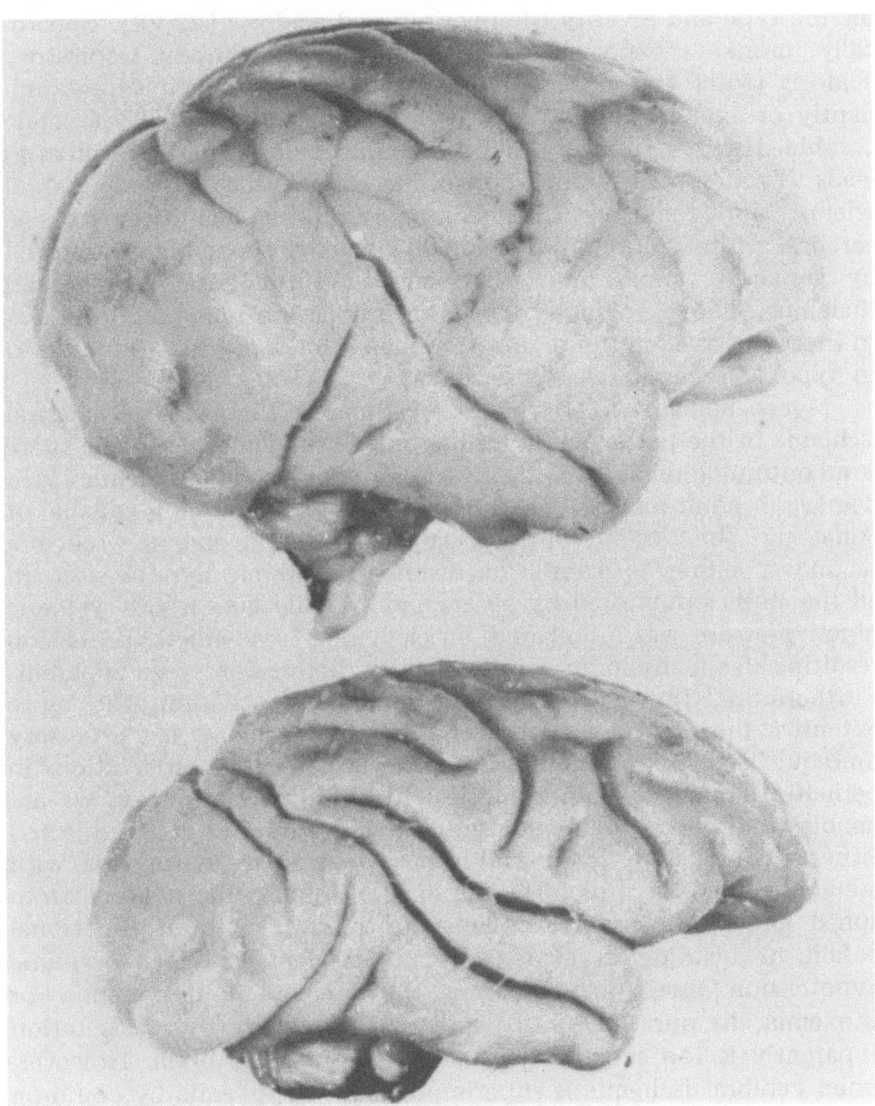

Figure 7. Gross brain specimens of newborn monkeys showing hypoxic-ischemic brain damage. The upper brain is that of a monkey subjected to prolonged partial asphyxia *in utero* at term and who survived the newborn period for 96 hours. Note the brain swelling with flattening of the convolutions and areas of softening with small vessel hemorrhage. The lower brain is that of a control newborn monkey, age six months, not previously subjected to intrauterine asphyxia. From Brann and Myers [28] with permission.

monkey is dependent on the severity of the systemic hypoxia and on the type and severity of superimposed acidosis [22,29]. Specifically, monkeys exposed to anoxemia with concurrent respiratory acidosis (total asphyxia) exhibit brain damage which is predominantly or exclusively restricted to brainstem structures. Hypoxemia combined with respiratory and metabolic acidosis (partial asphyxia) leads to widespread cerebral cortical necrosis with associated cerebral edema. Hypoxemia with little or no respiratory acidosis results in cerebral white matter injury. Finally, when hypoxemia is followed by anoxemia, brain injury is focused on the basal ganglia and thalamus. The topography of these lesions are remarkably similar to those observed in the brains of human infants previously subjected to hypoxic-ischemic stress (see above).

Myers appears to have underestimated the role of cerebral ischemia in the pathogenesis of hypoxic brain damage. Indeed, there is a continuing debate among investigators of hypoxic-ischemic brain damage in adult animals whether or not hypoxia alone is capable of damaging the brain without superimposing cerebral ischemia secondary either to arterial occlusion or systemic hypotension. In all the studies published by Myers and his colleagues where systemic blood pressure was monitored, an element of systemic hypotension resulting from hypoxic cardiovascular depression was apparent. Furthermore, the greater the degree of hypotension, the more extensive the neuropathology. That cerebral ischemia is a necessary prerequisite to hypoxic brain injury is supported by observations in perinatal animals of other species. In our own laboratory, we are unable to produce brain damage in newborn rats or dogs subjected either to anoxemia (asphyxia) or to progressive hypoxemia with metabolic acidosis [30-33]. Either the animals die acutely from apnea and cardiovascular collapse or recover without functional deficit or histological evidence of brain damage. When systemic hypotension does occur during the course of hypoxemia or anoxemia, its duration until death or to recovery by resuscitation apparently is too short to permanently injure the brain. However, when cerebral ischemia is superimposed on hypoxemia by common carotid artery occlusion, brain damage inevitably occurs [33]. These observations underscore the importance of cerebral ischemia in the pathogenesis of perinatal hypoxic-ischemic brain damage and explain the observation that such brain lesions occur only, or are accentuated at, arterial border zones (see above).

Over the past several years, my research colleagues and I have investigated a model of hypoxic-ischemic brain damage in the immature rat [33]. Our reasons for pursuing this line of research relate to the low cost of rats relative to perinatal animals of larger species, especially monkeys. In addition, rats are available in large numbers, which allows for statistical analysis of variables applied to the animals subjected to hypoxic-ischemic stress. The seven-day postnatal rat was chosen because at this stage of development the animal's brain is histologically similar to that of the 32-week gestation human fetus or newborn infant, that is, cerebral cortical neuronal layering is complete, the germinal matrix is involuting, and white matter as yet has undergone little myelination. The method to produce hypoxic-ischemic brain damage in these animals is based on the Levine preparation in the adult rat [34] and consists of unilateral (right) common carotid artery ligation followed four hours later by systemic hypoxia produced by the inhalation of 8% oxygen-balance nitrogen. The rat pups are capable of surviving this severity of hypoxia for three or more hours before an appreciable mortality occurs. Measurements of systemic physiological variables during the course of hypoxia reveal hypoxemia combined with hypocapnia produced by hyperventilation (Table 1). The hypocapnia compensates for the metabolic acidosis caused by lactacidemia, such that systemic pH does not change from the control value. Mean systemic blood pressure decreases during hypoxia to a low of 23 mm Hg (-23%) at two hours.

Table 1. Systemic Physiological Variables during Hypoxia in 7-Day-Old Postnatal Rats

Variable	Normoxia	Hypoxia (min)			
		20	60	120	180
Mean blood pressure (mm Hg)	30	27	25	23*	30
Heart rate (beats/min)	313	292	276	270	287
pO_2 (mm Hg)	98	45*	58*	57*	47*
pCO_2 (mm Hg)	44	23*	27*	23*	26*
Lactate (mmol/1)	0.9	7.8*	13.9*	13.8*	14.1*
pH	7.44	7.43	7.45	7.39	7.37

Hypoxia was produced by the inhalation of 8% oxygen-balance nitrogen at 37°C.
* Different from normoxia with $p < 0.05$.
Modified from Welsh et al. [35].

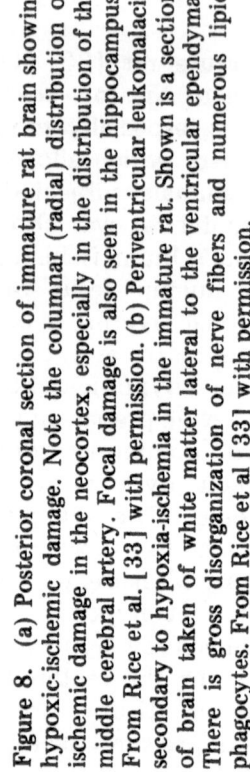

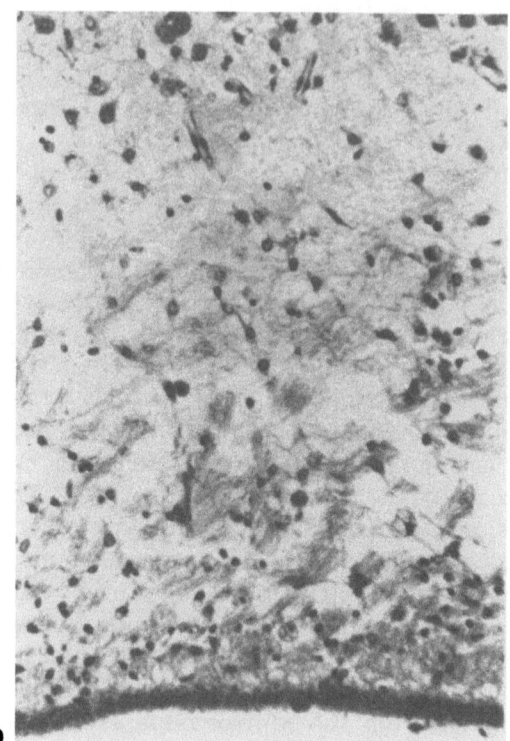

Figure 8. (a) Posterior coronal section of immature rat brain showing hypoxic-ischemic damage. Note the columnar (radial) distribution of ischemic damage in the neocortex, especially in the distribution of the middle cerebral artery. Focal damage is also seen in the hippocampus. From Rice et al. [33] with permission. (b) Periventricular leukomalacia secondary to hypoxia-ischemia in the immature rat. Shown is a section of brain taken of white matter lateral to the ventricular ependyma. There is gross disorganization of nerve fibers and numerous lipid phagocytes. From Rice et al [33] with permission.

Table 2.   Factors Governing the Topography of Hypoxic-Ischemic Brain Damage

A. Intrinsic Vulnerability
  1. Cellular: Neurons, glia, vessels
  2. Regional:
     Cerebral cortex: Layers 3 and 5 + 6
     Hippocampus: H 1 and H 3-5
     Cerebellum: Purkinje cell layer
B. Nature and duration of the systemic insult

Hypoxic-ischemic brain damage is a near universal finding in those immature rats surviving three hours of systemic hypoxia. By 16 to 50 hours of recovery, damage, restricted to the cerebral hemisphere ipsilateral to the common carotid artery occlusion, is observed in cerebral cortex, subcortical and periventricular white matter, striatum (basal ganglia) and hippocampus. Tissue injury takes the form of either selective neuronal necrosis (glia and blood vessels spared) or infarction (all elements destroyed). Neocortical damage is often laminar in distribution, with layers 3 and 5 + 6 bearing the brunt of injury, as in the adult. However, cortical damage also appears as columns of dead neurons adjacent to columns of preserved neurons oriented at right angles to the pial surface (Figure 8). This pattern of damage recently has been described in a premature infant subjected to repeated bouts of hypoxia–acidosis with hypotension and is proposed to be the early pathological lesion of ulegyria [36]. In the rat pups, there is also necorsis of subcortical and periventricular white matter, which originates in and spreads from so-called "myelinogenic foci," areas which are presumed to be the sites of origin of oligodendrocytes (Figure 8). The evolution of the ischemic cell change and the associated gliomesodermal reaction appears more rapid than what is found in adults. Thus, at least in the immature rat, hypoxic-ischemic damage involving cerebral cortex, white matter, and deep gray matter structure (basal ganglia and thalamus) can coexist in the same animal and, of necessity, results from the same hypoxic-ischemic stress. What effect age and variations in the systemic hypoxic stress (anoxia rather than hypoxia; hypoxia plus respiratory acidosis; hypoxia followed by anoxia) have on the severity and distribution of brain damage is yet unknown.

It is possible to conclude from experimentally induced perinatal hypoxic-ischemic brain damage that distinctive factors govern the topography of the pathological lesions (Table 2). First, there is an intrinsic vulnerability of the tissue to hypoxic-ischemic stress. At the cellular level, neurons appear more sensitive to hypoxia–ischemia, followed by glia (astrocytes, oligodendrocytes), followed by blood vessels (endothelia). There are also selective regional vulnerabilities which probably reflect underlying differences in anatomical maturation, metabolic requirements, and/or functional activities. Lastly, the nature and duration of the systemic insult contribute not only to the severity but also to the distribution of the pathological lesions; especially important here is the role of cerebral ischemia in the genesis of border zone injury. The manner by which various types of acidosis (respiratory, metabolic, combined) influence the ultimate pathology, as suggested by Myers [22,29], has yet to be confirmed.

THE CONTRIBUTION OF CEREBRAL EDEMA TO PERINATAL HYPOXIC-ISCHEMIC BRAIN DAMAGE

A well-known accompaniment to the brain damage that results from perinatal hypoxia–ischemia is cerebral edema [37–40]. Despite the close association between selective neuronal necrosis or infarction and brain swelling, it is not yet known whether edema is simply a by-product of tissue injury or whether edema actually leads to or accentuates brain damage. Based on studies primarily in adult animals and man, it has been assumed that the edema which arises from cerebral hypoxia–ischemia is of two types [41–43]. Initially, brain edema is cytotoxic in origin and results from failure of ionic pumping across the cell membrane with secondary intracellular accumulation of electrolytes and water. Vasogenic edema results from disruption of the blood–brain barrier with resultant free passage of large molecular weight substances from blood into brain parenchyma. Vasogenic edema temporally follows cytotoxic edema. Hypoxic-ischemic edema may aggravate brain damage, at least in adults, by increasing tissue volume in a non-distensible skull, thereby compromising the vascular compartment and decreasing cerebral perfusion below critical levels [42,44]. The role of edema in perinatal cerebral hypoxia–ischemia is not yet as well defined.

Brain edema is a common finding in autopsies of newborn human infants sustaining cerebral hypoxia–ischemia. Clifford [37] examined the brains of nine term infants who expired four to six hours following emergency cesarean section for placenta previa. The brains of seven of the nine infants demonstrated microscopic evidence of cerebral edema, as suggested clinically in two infants who exhibited bulging fontanels prior to death. Larroche [40] examined the brains of 15 full-term infants dying up to nine days postasphyxia and found swelling of the cerebral hemispheres with secondary uncal herniation in all 15. Pryse–Davis and Beard [38] performed 183 consecutive autopsies on infants 20 to 42 weeks gestational age. Brain swelling was noted in one third of the infants and was characterized by gyral flattening alone or gyral flattening in association with uncal grooving and/or cerebellar coning. Paradoxically, no consistent histological evidence of brain edema was identified by light microscopy. Anderson and Belton [39] measured sodium, potassium, and water contents in the brains of 16 severely asphyxiated infants, 14 of whom were full-term. Brain water content was increased over that of age-matched controls when survival exceeded 48 hours. Increased brain sodium and decreased brain potassium occurred in all infants regardless of the length of survival. Four infants had gross autopsy evidence of brain swelling, and one of these four exhibited cerebral cortical necrosis. Anderson and Belton [39] suggested that the water and electrolyte abnormalities present in the edematous brains represented early hypoxic-ischemic damage (necrosis), as the abnormalities were present even on the first day of postnatal life and appeared to precede the development of gross brain swelling. These published reports indicate that brain swelling is a prominent feature of human perinatal cerebral hypoxia–ischemia.

To ascertain the nature and time–course of the edema which accompanies perinatal hypoxic-ischemic brain damage, we performed a series of experiments in our animal model of perinatal hypoxic-ischemic brain damage [45]. Seven-day-old postnatal rats were lightly anesthetized with halothane during which time the right common carotid artery was irreversibly ligated. Four hours later, the animals were exposed to 8% oxygen-balance nitrogen at 37°C for up to three hours. During the course of hypoxia and recovery, the rat pups were decapitated; their brains were removed and analyzed for water content. During hypoxia, water content of the cerebral hemisphere ipsilateral to the arterial occlusion increased in near linear fashion to a maximum at three hours of hypoxia (Figure 9). Brain water content remained high during the first 24 hours of recovery, following which it steadily decreased to a level equal to that of the contralateral hemisphere at 72 hours. The increase in water content,

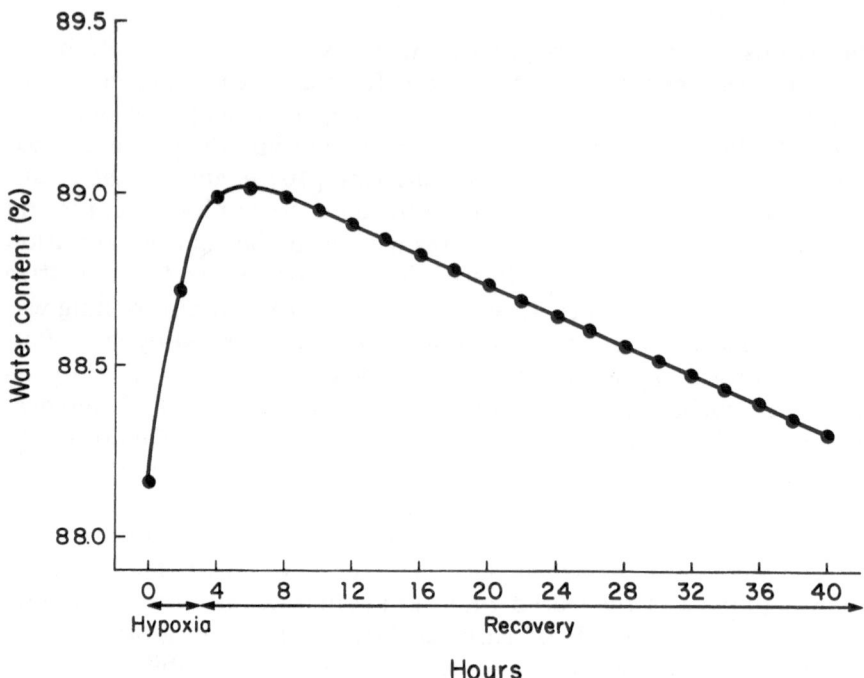

Figure 9. The time course of the edema which accompanies hypoxic-ischemic brain damage in the seven-day-old rat. The line depicts the computer-assisted best fit curve of cerebral hemispheric water content ipsilateral to the common carotid artery occlusion during and following cerebral hypoxia–ischemia. No increase in water content was noted in the contralateral cerebral hemisphere.

equivalent to cerebral edema, occurred in 100% of the animals and, thus, was comparable to the 92% incidence of histological alteration seen in the brains of these animals [33].

To assess the degree of hypoxic-ischemic injury to the blood-brain barrier, horseradish peroxidase (HRP) or Evan's blue dye was injected I.P. into seven-day-old rats from 0 to 48 hours of recovery from cerebral hypoxia–ischemia. Macroscopic (Evan's blue) or microscopic (HRP) staining of the ipsilateral cerebral hemisphere was seen in 30% and 89% of the brains, respectively, and the presence and extent of staining appeared uniform from 0 to 24 hours of recovery (Figures 10 and 11). As with histologically confirmed cerebral infarction, the HRP and Evan's blue staining was most prominent in the territory of the middle cerebral artery. The incidence of Evan's blue staining is comparable to the incidence of infarction (37%) in this region.

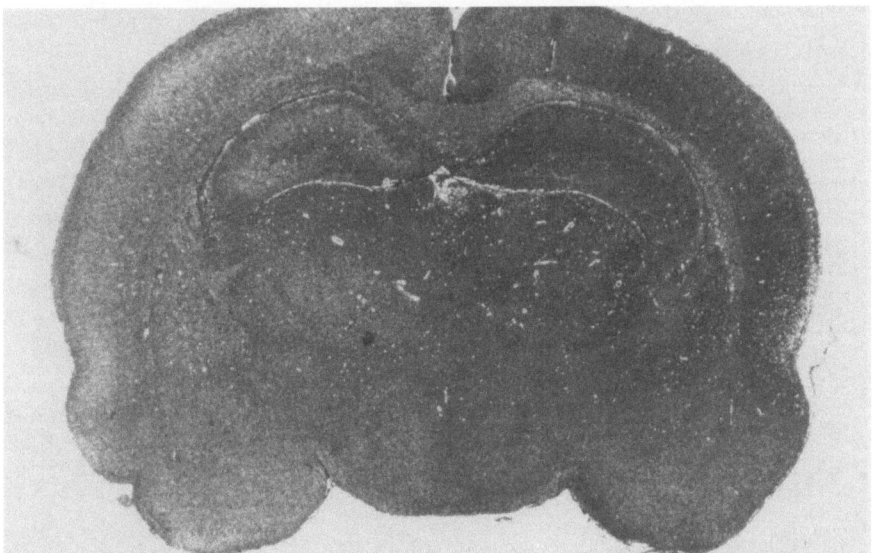

Figure 10. Representative coronal section of brain from a seven-day-old rat injected with horseradish peroxidase (HRP) 12 hours following cerebral hypoxia-ischemia. Note the moderately intense staining in the cerebral hemisphere ipsilateral to the common carotid artery occlusion (right side) compared to the contralateral hemisphere. Patchy areas of staining are apparent in cerebral cortex, which are oriented perpendicular to the pial surface. Staining is also prominent in hippocampus and thalamus.

The results of the investigation under discussion indicate that cerebral edema is an early and inevitable accompaniment to the brain damage that results from perinatal cerebral hypoxia–ischemia [28]. Both cytotoxic and vasogenic components of the edema are present and occur in association with and reflect the severity of cerebral injury. Thus, the findings are entirely consistent with those reported to occur in the brains of adult animals to similar hypoxic-ischemic stress [41,43,46]. What the study did not resolve was whether or not brain edema, whatever its form, contributes to or accentuates perinatal hypoxic-ischemic brain injury. However, evidence from separate experiments in our laboratory supports the notion that edema may contribute to the ultimate neuropathology. We have recently devised a technique to restore blood flow through the right common carotid artery in seven-day-old rats within 15 minutes of recovery from only two hours of hypoxia (previous neuropathological examinations were performed following three hours of hypoxia). Eleven

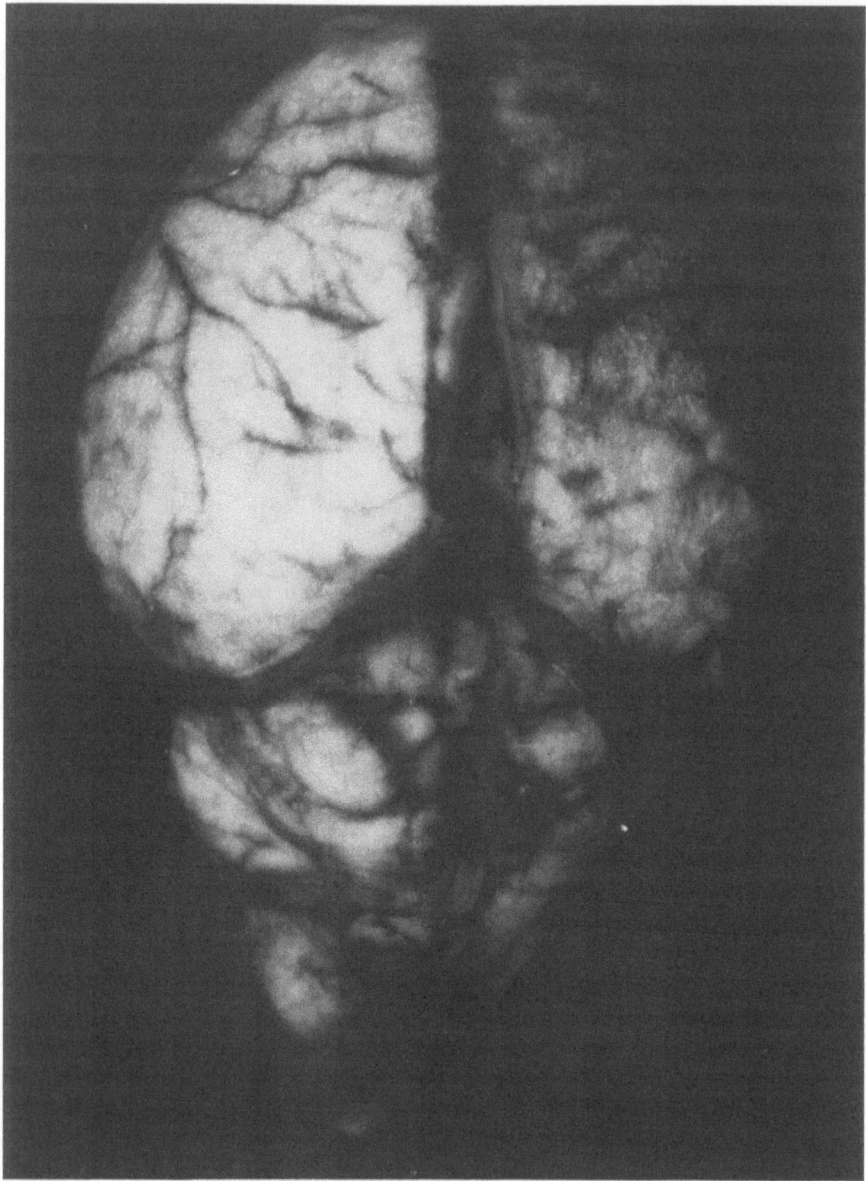

Figure 11. Brain of a seven-day-old rat injected with Evan's blue dye 24 hours following cerebral hypoxia–ischemia. Note the discoloration of the cerebral hemisphere ipsilateral to the common carotid artery occlusion (right side), especially in the distribution of the middle cerebral artery. The staining seen in the contralateral cerebral hemisphere is restricted to the pial blood vessels.

of 12 brains from animals with temporary arterial occlusion exhibited ipsilateral infarction determined by visual inspection at 30 days of postnatal age compared to only 1 of 12 brains in littermates with permanent ligations. Mean water content of the ipsilateral cerebral hemispheres in the temporarily ligated animals at four hours of survival posthypoxia was increased by 90% over that of hemispheres from animals with permanent ligations ($p < 0.01$). Presumably, release of the carotid artery ligature preferentially restored ipsilateral blood flow well above that of the permanently ligated animals; the greater perfusion pressure accentuated brain swelling and ultimate tissue damage.

CONCLUSIONS

The investigations described here demonstrate the susceptability of the immature brain to hypoxic-ischemic stress. Furthermore, the nature and distribution of the pathological reaction to hypoxia-ischemia adequate to produce tissue injury are well documented. Attention must now be focused on the response of the fetal and newborn brain to altered states of oxygenation and perfusion and on whether therapeutic intervention can prevent or minimize the neurological sequelae of perinatal hypoxia–ischemia.

REFERENCES

1. Little, W. J. On the influence of abnormal parturition, difficult labors, premature birth and asphyxia neonatorium on the mental and physical conditions of the child, especially in relation to deformities. *Lancet 2*:378–381, 1861.
2. Banker, B. Q., and Larroche, J. C. Periventricular leukomalacia of infancy. *Arch. Neurol. 7*:386–410, 1962.
3. Christiensen, E., and Melchoir, J. *Cerebral Palsy—A Clinical and Neuropathological Study, Clinics of Developmental Medicine*. Philadelphia: Spastics International Medical Publications, J. B. Lippincott Co., 1967.
4. Courville, C. B. In: *Birth and Brain Damage*, edited by M. F. Courville. Pasedena, 1971.
5. Malamud, N. An etiologic and diagnostic study of cerebral palsy. In *Selective Vulnerability of the Brain in Hypoxaemia*, edited by J. P. Schade and W. H. McMenemy. Philadelphia: F. A. Davis, 1963.
6. Vannucci, R. C., and Plum, F. Pathophysiology of perinatal hypoxic-ischemic brain damage. In: *Biology of Brain Dysfunction*, Vol. III, edited by G. E. Gaull. New York: Plenum Press, 1975.
7. Volpe, J. J. *Neurology of the Newborn*. Philadelphia: W. B. Saunders Co., 1981.

8. Brierley, J. B., Brown, A. W., Excell, B. J., and Meldrum, B. S. Brain damage in the rhesus monkey resulting from profound arterial hypotension. 1. Its nature, distribution and general physiological correlates. *Brain Res. 13*: 68-74, 1969.

9. Brierley, J. B., Meldrum, B. S., and Brown, A. W. The threshold and neuropathology of cerebral "anoxic-ischemic" cell change. *Arch Neurol. 29*:367-374, 1973.

10. Takashima, S., Armstrong, D. L., and Becker, L. E. Subcortical leukomalacia: Relationship to development of the cerebral sulcus and its vascular supply. *Arch. Neurol. 35*:470-472, 1978.

11. DeReuck, J. The human periventricular arterial blood supply and the anatomy of cerebral infarction. *Europ. Neurol. 5*:321-334, 1971.

12. DeReuck, J., Chattha, A. S., and Richardson, E. P. Pathogenesis and evolution of periventricular leukomalacia in infancy. *Arch Neurol. 27*:229-236, 1972.

13. Takashima, S., and Taraka, K. Development of cerebrovascular architecture and its relationship to periventricular leukomalacia. *Arch Neurol. 35*:11-16, 1978.

14. Borit, A., and Herndon, R. M. The fine structure of plaques fibromyeliniques in ulegyria in status marmoratus. *Acta Neuropath. 14*:304-308, 1970.

15. Malamud, N. Status marmoratus: A form of cerebral palsy following either birth injury or inflammation of the central nervous system. *J. Pediatr. 37*: 610-619, 1950.

16. Leech, R. W., and Alvord, E. C. Anoxic-ischemic encephalopathy in the human neonatal period. The significance of brain stem involvement. *Arch Neurol. 34*:109-113, 1977.

17. Schneider, H., Ballowitz, L., Schachinger, H., Hanefeld, F., and Droszus, J. U. Anoxic encephalopathy with predominant involvement of basal ganglia, brain stem and spinal cord in the perinatal period. *Acta Neuropathol. 32*:287-298, 1975.

18. Brierley, J. B. The influence of brain swelling, age, and hypotension upon the pattern of cerebral damage in hypoxia. In: *Proceedings of the 5th Congress of Neuropathology*, New York: Excepta Medica, 1966.

19. Hicks, S. P., Vacanaugh, M. C., and O'Brien, E. D. Effects of anoxia on the developing cerebral cortex in the rat. *Am. J. Pathol. 40*:615-628, 1962.

20. Jilek, L., Fischer, J., Krulich, L., et al. The reaction of the brain to stagnant hypoxia and anoxia during ontogeny. *Prog. Brain Res. 9*:113-131, 1964.

21. Windle, W. F. Brain damage at birth: Functional and structural modifications with time. *J. Am. Med. Assoc. 206*:1967-1972.

22. Myers, R. E. Experimental models of perinatal brain damage: Relevance to human pathology. In: *Intrauterine Asphyxia and the Developing Fetal Brain*, edited by L. Gluck. Chicago: Yearbook Medical Publishers, 1977.

23. Ranck, J. B., and Windle, W. F. Brain damage in the monkey, *Macaca mulatta*, by asphyxia neonatrum. *Exp. Neurol. 1*:130-154, 1959.

24. Windle, W. F. *Pysiology of the Fetus*. Springfield, Ill.: Charles C Thomas Co., 1971.

25. Faro, M. D., and Windle, W. F. Transneuronal degeneration in brains of monkeys asphyxiated at birth. *Exp. Neurol. 24*:38-53, 1969.

26. Myers, R. E., Beard, R., and Adamsons, K. Brain swelling in the newborn rhesus monkey following prolonged partial asphyxia. *Neurology 19*:1012-1018, 1969.

27. Seltzer, M. E., Myers, R. E., and Holstein, S. F. Prolonged partial asphyxia: Effects of fetal brain water and electrolytes. *Neurology* 22:732-737, 1972.
28. Brann, A. W., and Myers, R. E. Central nervous system findings in the newborn monkey following severe *in utero* partial asphyxia. *Neurology* 25:327-338, 1975.
29. Myers, R. E. Four patterns of perinatal brain damage and their conditions of occurrence in primates. In: *Advances in Neurology*, Vol. 10, edited by B. S. Meldrum and C. D. Marsden. New York: Raven Press, 1975.
30. Vannucci, R. C., and Duffy, T. E. Cerebral oxidative and energy metabolism of fetal and neonatal rats during anoxia and recovery. *Am. J. Physiol. 230*: 1269-1275, 1976.
31. Vannucci, R. C., and Duffy, T. E. Cerebral metabolism in newborn dogs during reversible asphyxia. *Ann. Neurol. 1*:528-534, 1977.
32. Vannucci, R. C., Nardis, E. E., Vannucci, S. J., et al. Tolerance of the perinatal brain to graded hypoxemia. *Neurology 30*:443-444, 1980.
33. Rice, J. E., Vannucci, R. C., and Brierley, J. B. The influence of immaturity on hypoxic-ischemic brain damage in the rat. *Ann. Neurol. 9*:131-141, 1981.
34. Levine, S. Anoxic-ischemic encephalopathy in rats. *Am. J. Pathol. 36*:1-17, 1960.
35. Welsh, F. A., Vannucci, R. C., and Brierley, J. B. Columnar alterations of NADH fluorescence during hypoxia-ischemia in immature rat brain. *J. Cereb. Blood Flow Metabol. 2*:221-228, 1982.
36. Norman, M. G. On the morphogenesis of ulegyria. *Acta. Neuropath. 53*: 331-332, 1981.
37. Clifford, S. H. The effects of asphyxia on the newborn infant. *J. Pediat. 18*: 567-578, 1941.
38. Pryse-Davis, J., and Beard, R. W. A necropsy study of brain swelling in the newborn with special reference to cerebellar herniation. *J. Pathol. 109*: 51-56.
39. Anderson, J. M., and Belton, N. R. Water and electrolyte abnormalities in the human brain after severe intrapartum asphyxia. *J. Neurol. Neurosurg. Psychiat. 37*:514-520, 1974.
40. Larroche, J. C. L. *Developmental Pathology of the Neonate*. New York: Elsevier Science Publishing Co., 1977.
41. Klatzo, I. Neuropathological aspects of brain edema. *J. Neuropathol. Exp. Neurol. 26*:1-14, 1967.
42. Katzman, R., Clasen, R., Klatzo, I., Meyer, J. S., Pappius, H. M., and Waltz, A. G. Report of joint committee for stroke resources: IV. Brain edema in stroke. *Stroke 8*:512-540, 1977.
43. O'Brien, M. D. Ischemic cerebral edema. A Review. *Stroke 10*:623-628, 1979.
44. Fishman, R. A. Brain edema. *N. Eng. J. Med. 293*:706-711, 1975.
45. McAfoos, G. L., and Vannucci, R. C. The nature and extent of cerebral edema in perinatal hypoxic-ischemic brain damage. Submitted to *Pediat. Res.*, 1983.
46. Ito, U., Ohno, K., Nakamura, R., Suganuma, F., and Inaba, Y. Brain edema during ischemia and after restoration of blood flow: Measurement of water, sodium, potassium content and plasma protein permeability. *Stroke 10*: 542-547, 1979.

CHAPTER 3

Current Concepts of Pathophysiology of Perinatal Intraventricular Hemorrhage

Jan Goddard-Finegold, M.D.

THE CLINICAL PROBLEM

The term perinatal intracranial hemorrhage now evokes from most pediatricians, neonatologists, neurologists, and pathologists the thought of intracerebral, periventricular, intraventricular hemorrhage (PIVH). PIVH occurs most commonly in premature newborns of less than 32 weeks gestational age, most of whom have suffered the respiratory distress syndrome [1-9]. Most affected babies have sustained some degree of perinatal asphyxia [10]. The newborns who are symptomatic usually deteriorate, either suddenly or gradually, within the first three days after birth with bulging fontanelles, abnormalities on neurologic examination, bloody spinal fluid, a greater than 10% decrease in hematocrit, hypoglychorrachia, hyperglycemia, hypotension, and manifestations of seizure activity [6,7,9].

These are the cardinal signs and symptoms of PIVH, but a significant proportion of affected infants exhibit only some of them, and a number of infants with hemorrhages are asymptomatic [6]. Two evaluations by computerized tomography (CT) of newborns of less than either 1500- or 1750-gm. birthweight revealed PIVH in 40 to 43% of the cases [1-6]. Twenty-five percent of the infants studied by Papile et al, who had PIVH on CT scans, were asymptomatic by

Perinatal Neurology and Neurosurgery. Edited by R. A. Thompson, J. R. Green, and S. D. Johnsen. Copyright © 1985 by Spectrum Publications, Inc.

clinical assessment at the time of the scans. At present, evaluation for hemorrhages is usually accomplished by bedside ultrasound examinations [11-15]. Ultrasound scans can be done as early as the first few hours after birth without having to transport the very fragile, often mechanically ventilated immature newborn.

One prospective evaluation of premature newborns, in which real-time ultrasound imaging of the brain was used to detect PIVH, revealed hemorrhages in 90% of babies less than 34 weeks gestational age [11]. A large percentage of these hemorrhages were documented early in the first postnatal day. The high incidence of hemorrhages in this study population has yet to be explained.

The respiratory distress syndrome has become a less frequent cause of neonatal mortality, and PIVH has taken its place as the major harbinger of neonatal death. In addition, it has become the most easily identified marker for serious brain insult in the perinatal period.

GRADES OF PIVH

The criteria for CT evaluation of severity of these lesions were devised by Papile in 1978 [6]. These grades of hemorrhage often conform to findings at autopsy, especially if the blood has not resolved by the time of death [10]. This scheme, which is now applied to ultrasound images and is widely used in neonatal nurseries, consists of the following classification:

Grade I: Hemorrhage which is subependymal only.
Grade II: Intraventricular hemorrhage with or without evidence of subependymal hemorrhage, without dilation of ventricle(s).
Grade III: Intraventricular hemorrhage with dilation of ventricle(s).
Grade IV: Intraventricular hamorrhage plus intraparenchymal hemorrhage.

Since the classification was published, progression of lesions from Grades I and II to Grades III and IV over periods of hours to days has been documented by serial scans [14]. This progression may be reflected clinically in what has been termed the "stuttering" or "saltatory" course, during which newborns have multiple episodes of clinical deterioration instead of a single catastrophic event [7,9].

SEQUELAE

Three recent follow-up studies indicate that the degree of neurological impairment following PIVH is related to the severity of the hemorrhages and that about 65% of the survivors of moderate to severe hemorrhages (Grades III and IV) will have posthemorrhagic hydrocephalus [16-18]. In Williamson's study, over 50% of the survivors of symptomatic and CT-documented PIVH had functional neurological impairments [18]. These impairments included blindness, spastic di- and quadripareses, hearing loss, seizures, mental retardation, and delayed language and fine motor skills. In the follow-up study of Papile, major neurological handicaps were present in 75% of infants one to five years following documentation of severe hemorrhage [17].

PATHOLOGY

The lesions were first extensively described in autopsy studies. Larroche, Leech and Kohnen, and Towbin showed that the majority of hemorrhages in the premature newborns (up to 87%) originated in the germinal matrix layer (GML)—the zone of periventricular germinal cells still present in the premature newborn [5,8,19]. This zone of cells is most prominent ventrally in the human, over the head of the caudate nucleus, and becomes distinctly less prominent by term. Some germinal cells persist into the first few months of life, however, and migrating cells, or "germinal rests," are not uncommon findings in brains of infants dying before six months of age [20]. Most neuroblasts are thought to have migrated prior to the third trimester, so that later GML cells are probably precursors to astrocytes, oligodendroglial cells, and ependymal cells [21].

It has been shown in human autopsy studies that there is a regional predisposition to hemorrage which seems to be dependent upon gestational age [4]. Infants born at less than 28 weeks gestation have more hemorrhages in that part of the GML overlying the body of the caudate nucleus; infants of greater than 28 weeks gestational age have more hemorrhages at the head of the caudate near the foramen of Monro. These findings may reflect the pattern of maturation and involution of the GML.

While intraventricular hemorrhage most often originates in the GML, it can also originate from the highly vascular choroid plexus. In fact, the incidence of choroid plexus hemorrhage may have been underestimated in past studies. Both Larroche and Leech and Kohnen reported an incidence of choroid plexus hemorrhage of from 4 to 10% in premature newborns [5,19]. However, a recent study by Armstrong utilizing serial sections has shown that (1) the choroid plexus is a site of origin of hemorrhage in up to 41% of premature newborns with PIVH, and (2)GML and choroid plexus hemorrhages may occur simultaneously [22]. Choroid plexus hemorrhages may not have been recognized in many cases in the past because GML hemorrhage can obscure the site of origin of hemorrhage in the choroid or the tela choroidea. It has also been shown that when term infants have PIVH, which is rare but has been more frequently recognized recently due to the diagnostic capabilities of CT and ultrasound scanning [23,24], these hemorrhages are more likely to originate from the choroid plexus than from the GML [25].

The fact that sites of hemorrhages vary with gestational age may be a reflection of (1) differing vascular structural maturities, (2) variations in vascular regulatory mechanisms, (3) susceptibility to different physiological hemodynamic stresses, or (4) heterogeneous metabolic needs which are age dependent. The advantage to knowing the details of pathogenesis of hemorrhages obviously lies in their application toward means of prevention.

An interesting aspect of the pathology has been brought to light recently. It has been assumed from CT scan studies that rupture of the ventricular ependyma and extravasation of blood into periventricular white matter is the sequence of events which yields a Grade IV hemorrhage. This probably does occur, but very rarely. Flodmark et al documented intraparenchymal hemorrhage in 21 infants at autopsy; 20 of these were secondary hemorrhages into areas of periventricular leukomalacia (PVL) [10,26]. Only one hemorrhage was judged to be a direct extention from the ventricles. Armstrong et al question whether extension of blood from the ventricles ever occurs into normal white matter [22]. Whether large PIVH can cause enough compression of the surrounding white matter to actually induce infarction in that area has not been determined.

PATHOGENESIS

That very premature infants are subjected to asphyxial and hemodynamic stresses in the immediate perinatal period which predispose the germinal matrix layer (GML) and the white matter to periods of both under- and overperfusion is a hypothesis currently being evaluated in numerous animal and human studies. These studies are yielding information about the pathogenesis of PIVH and about reactions of the immature cerebrovasculature. Nevertheless, the events which underlie the ultimate disruption of vascular integrity in either the GML or the choroid plexus are still not entirely clear. Early studies were based upon autopsy examinations and implicated rupture or thrombosis of the terminal vein or its branches as the mechanisms finally responsible for hemorrhages [3,5, 18,19]. However, in 1975, Hambleton and Wigglesworth implicated the capillaries, the arteriolaer–capillary junctions, or the capillary–venule junctions as the most likely sources of hemorrhage [4]. They injected barium solutions at pressures near 80 mm Hg into the carotid arteries at autopsy and produced leaks of barium in the GML capillary plexus. In no instance was the terminal vein ruptured. When barium was injected into the jugular veins, leaks also occurred in the GML in one instance. From these studies they raised the hypothesis that increases in arterial or venous pressures could cause GML hemorrhages under conditions in which such increases might be transmitted to the vessels of the GML [4].

More recently, Lou et al have shown that a pressure-passive situation is present in the fetal sheep brain when asphyxia has rendered autoregulatory mechanisms ineffective [28]. Human newborns seem to exhibit the same loss of autoregulation after only moderate asphyxia [29]. The loss of autoregulation under similar circumstances has been documented in adult animals and humans [30]. Does autoregulation have to be absent, however, for increases in blood pressure to be reflected in the GML or the choroid plexus? In some cases, probably not, since autoregulation refers to those mechanisms that maintain constant cerebral blood flow (CBF) by variations in cerebrovascular resistance in response to changes in systemic arterial blood pressures over a fairly well defined range. Thus, blood pressure increases or decreases which are very rapid and those which are over or under the autoregulatory range may be directly reflected in the cerebral vasculature.

Another hypothesis raised by Hambleton and Wigglesworth is that hemorrhage might be more likely to occur in the GML if that area were to be reperfused, or hyperperfused, after a period of ischemia [4]. Postischemic hyperperfusion (the luxury perfusion syndrome) has been documented in adult animals and humans [31]. Unfortunately, studies which could directly test these hypotheses cannot be accomplished safely in the newborn human. Multiple examinations of GML hemorrhages and choroid plexus hemorrhages would have to be done, and their relationships to blood flow patterns would have to be assessed.

ANIMAL STUDIES

The way to accomplish these tasks is to use an animal which can withstand extensive hemodynamic monitoring and which will have PIVH under experimental conditions that is as similar as possible to that seen in the human preterm infant. To fulfill the latter, the animal has to have at least one major index of cerebral immaturity—a substantial germinal matrix zone. All of these criteria have been met by two animal models to date, the fetal sheep and the term beagle pup from one to three days of age [32,33]. In addition, the fetal rabbit has been shown to have spontaneous PIVH [34]. The most current experiments which have increased our knowledge of the pathogenesis of these lesions have come from studies in the fetal sheep and the newborn beagle. These animals have also been suitable for studies of regional cerebral blood flow.

The hypothesis of Hambleton and Wigglesworth was tested in both the fetal lamb and the newborn beagle pup. Reynolds et al subjected lambs at 58 to 85 days gestation to asphyxia plus increases in arterial and venous blood pressures. Asphyxia was induced by underventilation and supply of only 8 to 12% FiO_2 or by partial occlusion of the maternal aorta; arterial hypertension was induced by producing hypovolemia with maternal-fetal transfusion, or by intra-vascular injections of noradrenaline [33]. Raised venous pressure was achieved by transient superior vena caval obstruction by an adjust-able silicone snare. Significant peri- and intraventricular hemorrhages were produced in fetal lambs subjected to asphyxia plus raised arterial or venous pressures and in lambs subjected to raised arterial pressure alone. It is noteworthy that hemorrhages appeared to be of both capillary and capillary–venule origin in the GML; bleeding associated with increases in intravascular pressure were mainly from the choroid plexus. Animals subjected to asphyxia alone or to raised venous pressure alone did not have an increased incidence of hemorrhage when compared to control fetuses.

Goddard et al produced subependymal germinal matrix and intra-ventricular hemorrhages in two of five beagle pups from 24 to 72 hours of age subjected to rapid and severe increases in CO_2 tensions [32]. Four other pups rendered gradually moderately hypercarbic did not have hemorrhages. It has been shown that the newborn pup will increase cerebral blood flow in response to increases in pCO_2 [35,36]. Cerebral blood flows were not quantitated in these initial studies, but the increases in pCO_2 in the pups that hemorrhaged were quite dramatic and may have been associated with substantial increases in blood flow to both GML and the choroid plexus, especially since the two pups with hemorrhages were found to have had arterial blood pressures during the hypercarbia which were significantly higher than those of the other pups in the series [32].

Further studies in the same laboratory showed that the newborn beagle would also have PIVH when rendered rapidly, but moderately hypertensive by intravenous infusions of phenylephrine hydrochloride [37]. Arterial blood pressures in these pups increased from 53.68 ± 1.10 mm Hg to 81.92 ± 5.14 mm Hg [37]. As in the studies of Reynolds, while some hemorrhages originated in the GML, most came from the choroid plexus. These studies were followed by those in which hypovolemic hypotension was induced by phlebotomy so that arterial blood pressure decreased by 45 to 50%. Five minutes after the onset of hypotension, the blood volume was rapidly reinfused. Three of four animals so treated had significant PIVH with origins in the GML, the choroid plexus, the tela choroidea, and subependymal sites not in the GML [38]. During reinfusion, these pups experienced arterial blood pressures greater than their baseline pressures. Pups given saline to induce a hypervolemic state had elevations in jugular venous pressures with some hemorrhages in the germinal matrix without intraventricular extensions; pups rendered hypovolemic for the initial five-minute period, but not reinfused, had no significant hemorrhages in any of the sites [38].

Subsequent evaluations of this same protocol by Ment et al also resulted in PIVH in 75% of the pups [39]. In addition, CBF was assessed by autoradiographic methods at one hour after reperfusion in these pups and was found to be significantly increased when compared to control animals.

Goddard-Finegold and Michael quantitated regional cerebral blood flow using radioactive microspheres three times in each of nine pups subjected to hypovolemia plus rapid volume reinfusion [40]. Three of the nine pups had microscopically visible intraventricular hemorrhages. While the initial hypothesis was that this protocol was producing hemorrhage during reperfusion after a period of cerebral ischemia induced during the hypovolemia, in fact, ischemia could not be documented. Instead, blood flow increases to all regions sampled were documented during the acute, severe hypotension, and during the reperfusion blood flows increased even further [40].

The authors offered the following hypothesis to account for these findings. Pups not in cardiogenic shock may utilize peripheral and central mechanisms to compensate for the decreased cardiac output. These include cerebral vasodilatation, baroreceptor enhancement of sympathetic stimulation and carotid chemoreceptor-mediated hyperventilation, peripheral vasoconstriction, increased bronchiolar tone, increased pulmonary vascular resistance, increased adrenal steroid and catecholamine secretion, increased blood pressure, and bradycardia. Additional early compensatory mechanisms would lead to increased intravascular fluid volume and would effect a shunting of blood volume initially to the brain and myocardium during the hypovolemia. Thus, initially, ischemia of the brain would be averted. The replenishment of blood volume rapidly to this system, while the peripheral vasoconstriction and cerebral vasodilatory responses were still in force, would result in an increase in volume and flow in the circuits already being perfused (that is, the brain). If the vessels could not handle these rapid increases in blood volume and flow, hemorrhage might result [40].

There is evidence to indicate that the vessels of the GML are not structurally mature. They lack elastin and collagen, and venous channels make direct anastomoses at right angles to capillaries [4,41]. These features would tend to predispose to rupture.

Further studies of blood flow in the GML itself by Pasternak et al indicate that it is a "low-flow" area [42]. Its blood flows are similar to those of the periventricular white matter. Takashima and Tanaka have shown that in the human the GML is a border-zone region between the striate and medullary arteries and the deep venous drainage system [43]. Similarly, the periventricular white matter is a border-zone between the ventriculofugal and ventriculo-petal arterial supplies in the newborn. Two questions arise: (1) Is the GML, as a low-flow structure with its border-zone vascular structure more susceptible and more likely to be subjected to ischemia? and, (2) Because of its low-flow nature and its structure, is it incapable of adjusting to rapid increases in flow?

One way of answering these questions would be to determine repeated flow values in the GML during changes in systemic blood pressure and cardiac output. In this way, its ability to adjust to changes in blood pressure could be assessed. Unfortunately, the GML is too small for flow evaluation by the radioactive microsphere technique, and with autoradiography flows can only be determined one time in the same experimental animal. While autoregulation has been shown to be present in the 2- to 13-day-old dog [44,45], it has not yet been substantiated in the 1- to 2-day-old pup, or in the GML, and the question of whether the GML is being subjected to flows which are substantially different from those in other parts of the brain during hypovolemia or asphyxia has not been answered.

Pasternak has shown, however, that even at steady state, blood flow and glucose utilization in the GML of the newborn beagle pup are heterogeneous [46]. At term, blood flow and glucose utilization are low to the posterior GML, higher to GML between caudate and ependymal anterior to caudate, and highest to the anterior tip of the germinal matrix. The outer rim of the GML receives higher blood flow than the interior. The posterior-anterior gradient for both cerebral blood flow and glucose utilization appears to parallel the direction of involution of the GML.

Other studies, while not focusing primarily upon the production of hemorrhages, have nevertheless provided new information about how various physiological changes affect blood flow and metabolism in the immature brain.

Ashwal has shown that the fetal lamb responds to asphyxia and hypoxia by increasing CBF, a finding also supported by the work of Lou [27,28,47]. This response has also been documented in adult animals and man during hypoxia, early asphyxia, and anemia [48-51]. Tweed has shown that the fetal lamb preserves blood flow to the brain during moderate hypovolemic hypotension when compared to other organs, but does not increase its brain blood flow above steady state (in fact, CBF decreases mildly) [52]. Sola et al evaluated cerebral blood flow in newborn lambs subjected to a 50% decrease in blood volume for 90 minutes [53]. After 30 minutes of hypovolemia, maintenance of or increases in CBF compared to steady-state flow were present in those lambs surviving the hemorrhage for up to 90 minutes. However, in lambs not surviving as long as 90 minutes, CBF at 30 minutes was decreased by almost 50% compared to steady state. In Laptook's studies, newborn piglets subjected to asphyxia alone had increases in CBF, and piglets subjected to hypovolemic hypotension plus asphyxia were not able to maintain baseline CBF [54]. Piglets at five days of age subjected to hypovolemic hypotension for 24 minutes, during which systemic blood pressure was reduced by greater than 50%, had decreased cerebral blood flow to cerebrum and cerebellum at 10, 17, and 24 minutes [55]. However, increases in flow to the brain stem were evident in the piglets by 24 minutes. In Camp's study of hypoxic and hyperoxic 2- to 13-day-old mongrel pups, blood flow was constant during moderate hypotension (with blood pressure decreased by 20%) for fifteen minutes and during reperfusion over fifteen minutes [44]. All cerebral blood flow for the hypoxic puppies was higher than those of the hyperoxic puppies. Hernandez subjected anesthetized and paralyzed puppies up to one week of age to asphyxia by clamping the hoses to the endotracheal tube and turning off the ventilator for

five minutes [56]. Blood flow to the cortical structures fell dramatically after five minutes, while brain stem flow increased. The initial
blood flow responses to the asphyxia were not evaluated, but hemodynamic responses in the first 90 seconds of asphyxia included
marked tachycardia and moderate hypertension. Bucciarelli has
added data complementary to that obtained from studies of early
asphyxia and hypoxia by showing in perinatal goats that CBF
increases during acute acidosis [57].

NEW DIRECTIONS

These studies indicate that fetal and newborn animals have
sophisticated systemic and cerebral vascular responses to changes in
blood gas tensions, blood volume, blood pressure, and hematocrit.
They also indicate that the exact circumstances of experimental
protocol must be kept in mind when drawing conclusions about
these responses because variables such as duration and degree of
insult, species, and gestational or postnatal age of the animal may
affect the results.

While a hyperemic compensatory response to early onset, severe
hypovolemia has been shown to be present in the newborn, one- to
three-day-old beagle, the same response is not evident in hypoxic or
hypoxic pups that are ten days older and are subjected to more
moderate, but sustained, hypovolemia [40,44]. After ten minutes of
severe hypovolemia in piglets, the blood flow to the brain blood is
compromised [55]. If hypovolemia is instituted when piglets have
been asphyxiated, cerebral blood flow decreases; when newborn
piglets are subjected to asphyxia alone, blood flow increases initially
[54]. While cerebral blood flow responses have not been gauged in a
large number of human babies, Lou has shown that a pressure
passive response does exist in asphyxiated human newborns
[29]. Others have shown that initial hemodynamic responses of
newborn premature humans to asphyxia include at least early elevations in systemic blood pressure [58]. Early compensatory
responses to asphyxia or hypotension might be essential to preservation of brain function under many circumstances. During the birth of
an infant, increases in blood pressure and cerebral vasodilatory
responses to hypoxia and hypercapnia may ensure continuous
blood supply to the brain during cord compression or prolonged
passage through the vaginal canal. With normal vessels and
supporting structures and at least minimal clotting mechanisms, the

periventricular regions and choroid plexus of the term infant may be very little affected by these increases. On the other hand, even small changes in perfusion pressure and flow to the immature GML or the choroid plexus vasculature may stress their structural integrity. That plus inadequate clotting mechanisms put the asphyxiated and extensively resuscitated premature newborn at high risk for hemorrhage.

Premature infants are also at risk for other events that increase intravascular pressures. Mechanical ventilation and continuous end-expiratory pressures, as well as pneumothorax, cause increases in venous pressures [59,60]. Rapid closure of patent ductus arteriosus (PDA) is associated with increases in arterial pressures and may be associated with an increased risk of PIVH [61,62].

Premature newborns are also at risk for cerebral ischemia. PDA itself has been shown to enforce by its left to right shunt a "steal" of blood from cerebral arteries [63]. Also, with prolongation of asphyxia or hypovolemia, the early compensatory responses are compromised by acidosis and cardiac failure. The infant may suffer loss of cerebral autoregulation and perfusion with or without complete cardiac arrest. Successful resuscitation during cerebral ischemia may purposefully increase systemic and cerebral perfusion and flow, but may lead to hemorrhage in or near previously ischemic areas of brain which cannot withstand reperfusion.

Thus, the physician is caught in a potentially inescapable cycle. He must treat asphyxia and impending shock, yet, he has no way at present to gauge what has already happened or what will happen in the cerebral circulation of the newborn patient at the time he is making the most crucial clinical decisions. He knows that both underperfusion and overperfusion of the immature brain are deleterious, and he wants to maintain a physiological environment in which autoregulation can continue to function.

Clearly, noninvasive, continuous cerebral flow and function monitoring is a goal for the ideal future. The use of Doppler ultra-sound and the calculation of "pulsatility indices" for anterior cerebral artery flow are bringing us closer to this goal, but these methods are not easily applied, are not continuous, are not clearly safe, and are limited in being only applicable via fontanelles [64]. In the interim, while technology is progressing toward solution of this problem, while the solutions to premature labor are being discovered, and while the pathophysiology of hemorrhagic and ischemic lesions of the brain is being more firmly elucidated, prophylactic measures to prevent PIVH are being studied. If these prove successful, they may allow high-risk premature infants the chance to recover from initial physiological maladjustments and to combat other problems of prematurity without incurring PIVH.

Currently, studies of a sedating agent (phenobarbital), a capillary-stabilizing drug, ethamsylate, (Dicynene) and a vasoactive agent, indomethacin, (Indocin) are being carried out in newborn animals and humans. Conflicting results have been obtained in two clinical studies of phenobarbital [65,66]. One other study has shown its efficacy in diminishing arterial blood pressure peaks in newborns by decreasing their spontaneous motor activity [67]. Ethamsylate has been shown by Morgan et al to decrease the incidence of Grade I and II hemorrhages in one trial in human premature newborns in Great Britain [68]. Ment et al are continuing their studies of indomethacin, the prostaglandin synthetase inhibitor used to effect closure of patent ductus arteriosus. They have found a significantly reduced incidence of PIVH in beagle pups given indomethacin prior to hypovolemic hypotension followed by rapid reperfusion [69]. Indomethacin has been shown to reduce resting CBF in adult baboons and to mute the effects of changes in pCO_2 on CBF without altering autoregulation [70]. Side effects of indomethacin include severe inhibition of blood clotting mechanisms especially platelet adhesivity [71]. Carefully controlled clinical trials must be completed prior to its routine for prophylaxis against PIVH in nurseries.

Further studies are needed to assess the effects of agents such as those upon newborn cerebrovascular responses to pO_2 and pCO_2 changes, autoregulation, metabolism, and clotting mechanisms. With the accomplishment of these and other goals for better basic understanding of cerebral physiology in the premature and term newborn infant, we will be in a better position in the future to prevent the neurological handicaps which now result from brain damage in the neonatal period.

REFERENCES

1. Ahmann, P. A., Lazzara, A., Dykes, F. D., et al. Intraventricular hemorrhage in the high-risk preterm infant: incidence and outcome. *Ann. Neurol.* 7: 118-124, 1980.
2. Clark, C. E., Clyman, R. I., Roth, R. S., et al. Risk factor analysis of intraventricular hemorrhage in low birth weight infants. *J. Pediatr.* 99:625-628, 1981.
3. Cole, V. W., Durbin, G. M., Olaffson, A., et al. Pathogenesis of intraventricular hemorrhage in newborn infants. *Arch. Dis. Child.* 79:722-728, 1974.

4. Hambleton, G., and Wigglesworth, J. S. Origin of intraventricular hemorrhage in the preterm infant. *Arch Dis. Child. 51*:651-659, 1976.
5. Larroche, J. C. Hemorrhages cerebrales intraventriculares chez le premature. I. Anatomie et physiopathologie. *Biol. Neonate 7*:36-56, 1974.
6. Papile, L. A., Burstein, J., Burstein, R., et al. Incidence and evolution of subependymal and intraventricular hemorrhage: a study of infants with birth weights less than 1500 grams. *J. Pediatr. 92*:529-534, 1978.
7. Tarby, T. J., and Volpe, J. J. Intraventricular hemorrhage in the premature infant. *Pediatric Clinics of North America 29*:1077-1104, 1982.
8. Towbin, A. Cerebral intraventricular hemorrhage and subependymal matrix infarction in the fetus and premature newborn. *Am. J. Path. 52*:121-139, 1968.
9. Volpe, J. J. Neonatal intraventricular hemorrhage. *New Engl. J. Med. 304*: 886-890, 1981.
10. Flodmark, O., Becker, L. E., Harwood-Nash, D. C., et al. Correlation between computed tomography and autopsy in premature and full-term neonates that have suffered perinatal asphyxia. *Radiology 137*:93-103, 1980.
11. Bejar, R., Curbelo, V., Coen, R. W., et al. Diagnosis and follow-up of intraventricular and intracerebral hemorrhages by ultrasound studies of infant's brain through the fontanelles and sutures. *Pediatrics 66*:661-673, 1980.
12. Johnson, M. L., Mack, L. A., Rumack, C. M., et al. B-Mode echoencephalography in the normal and high risk infant. *Am. J. Radiol. 133*:375-381, 1979.
13. Johnson, M. L., Rumack, C. M., McAnnes, E. J., et al. Detection of neonatal intracranial hemorrhage utilizing real-time and static ultrasound. *J. Clin. Ultrasound 9*:427-433, 1981.
14. Shankaran, S., Slovis, T. L., Bedard, M. P., et al. Sonographic classification of intracranial hemorrhage. A prognostic indicator of mortality, morbidity, and short-term neurologic outcome. *J. Pediatr. 100*:469-475, 1982.
15. Silverboard, G., Horder, M. H., Ahmann, P. A., et al. Reliability of ultrasound in diagnosis of intracerebral hemorrhage and posthemorrhagic hydrocephalus: comparison with computerized tomography. *Pediatrics 66*:507-514, 1980.
16. Krishnamoorthy, K. S., Shannon, D. C., DeLong, G. R., et al. Neurologic sequelae in the survivors of neonatal intraventricular hemorrhage. *Pediatrics 64*:233-237, 1979.
17. Papile, L. A., Munsick-Bruno, G., and Schaefer, A. The relationship of cerebral intraventricular hemorrhage and early childhood neurologic handicaps. In: *Syllabus, The Second Special Ross Laboratories Conference on Perinatal Intracranial Hemorrhage. Vol. II*, edited by J. Lucey, 1982.
18. Williamson, W. D., Desmond, M. M., Wilson, G. S., et al. Early neurodevelopmental outcome of low birth weight infants surviving neonatal intraventricular hemorrhage. *J. Perinat. Med. 10*:34-40, 1982.
19. Leech, R. W., and Kohnen, P. Subependymal and intraventricular hemorrhages in the newborn. *Am. J. Path. 77*:465-475, 1974.
20. Friede, R. L. *Developmental Neuropathology*. New York: Springer-Verlag, 1980.
21. Dobbing, J., and Sands, J. Timing of neuroblast multiplication in developing human brain. *Nature 226*:639-640, 1970.

22. Armstrong, D. L., Goddard, J., Schwartz, M., et al. Another look at the pathology of intraventricular hemorrhage. In: *Ross Symposium on Perinatal Intracranial Hemorrhage*, edited by J. Lucey, 1980.
23. Chaplin, E. R., Goldstein, G. W., and Norman, D. Neonatal seizures, intracerebral hematoma, and subarachnoid hemorrhage in full-term infants. *Pediatrics 63*:812-815, 1979.
24. Palma, P. A., Miner, M. E., Morriss, F. H., et al. Intraventricular hemorrhage in the neonate born at term. *Am. J. Dis. Child. 133*:941-944, 1979.
25. Donat, J. F., Okazaki, H., Kleinberg, F., et al. Intraventricular hemorrhages in full-term and premature infants. *Mayo Clin. Proc. 53*:437-441, 1978.
26. Armstrong, D. L., and Norman, M. G. Preiventricular leukomalacia in neonates. Complications and sequelae. *Arch. Dis. Child. 49*:367-375, 1974.
27. Ashwal, S., Majcher, J. S., Vain, N., et al. Patterns of fetal lamb regional cerebral blood flow during and after prolonged hypoxia. *Pediatr. Res. 14*: 1104-1110, 1980.
28. Lou, H. C., Lassen, N. A., Tweed, W. A., et al. Pressure passive cerebral blood flow and breakdown of the blood-brain barrier in experimental fetal asphyxia. *Acta Paediatr. Scand. 68*:57-63, 1979.
29. Lou, H. C., Lassen, N. A., and Friis-Hansen, B. Impaired autoregulation of cerebral blood flow in the distressed newborn infant. *J. Pediatr. 94*:118-121, 1979.
30. Harper, A. M. General physiology of the cerebral circulation. *Internat. Anes. Clin. 7*:473, 1969.
31. Lassen, N. A. The luxury-perfusion syndrome and its possible relation to acute metabolic acidosis localized within the brain. *Lancet 2*:1113-1115, 1966.
32. Goddard, J., Lewis, R. M., Alcala, H., et al. Intraventricular hemorrhage—an animal model. *Biol. Neonate 37*:39-52, 1980.
33. Reynolds, M. L., Evans, C. A. N., Reynolds, E. O. R., et al. Intracranial haemorrhage in the preterm sheep fetus. *Early Human Devel. 3*(2):163-186, 1979.
34. Lorenzo, A. V., Welch, K., and Conner, S. Spontaneous germinal matrix and intraventricular hemorrhage in prematurely born rabbits. *J. Neurosurg. 56*: 404-410, 1982.
35. Cavazzuti, M., and Duffy, T. E. Regulation of local cerebral blood flow in normal and hypoxic newborn dogs. *Ann. Neurol. 11*:247-257, 1982.
36. Hernandez, M. J., Brennan, R. W., Vannucci, R. C., et al. Cerebral blood flow and oxygen consumption in the newborn dog. *Am. J. Physiol. 234*: R209-R215, 1978.
37. Goddard, J., Lewis, R. M., Armstrong, D., et al. Moderate, rapidly induced hypertension as a cause of intraventricular hemorrhage in the newborn beagle model. *J. Pediatr. 96*:1057-1060, 1980.
38. Goddard-Finegold, J., Armstrong, D., and Zeller, R. S. Intraventricular hemorrhage following volume expansion after hypovolemic hypotension in the newborn beagle. *J. Pediatr. 100*:796-799, 1982.
39. Ment, L. R., Stewart, W. B., Duncan, C. C., et al. Beagle puppy model of intraventricular hemorrhage. *J. Neurosurg. 57*:219-222, 1982.
40. Goddard-Finegold, J. and Michael, L. H. Cerebral blood flow and experimental intraventricular hemorrhage. *Pediatr. Res.*, *18*:7-11, 1984.

41. Haruda, F., and Blanc, W. A. The structure of intracerebral arteries in premature infants and the autoregulation of cerebral blood flow. *Ann. Neurol.* *10*:303, 1981.
42. Pasternak, J. F., Groothuis, D. R., Fisher, J. M., et al. Regional cerebral blood flow in the newborn beagle pup: the germinal matrix is a "low flow" structure. *Pediatr. Res. 16*:499-503, 1982.
43. Takashima, J., and Tanaka, K. Microangiography and vascular permeability of the subependymal matrix in the premature infant. *Can. J. Neurol. Sci.* *5*:45-50, 1978.
44. Camp, D., Kotagal, U. R., and Kleinman, L. I. Preservation of cerebral autoregulation in the unanesthetized hypoxemic newborn dog. *Brain Res.* *241*:207-213, 1982.
45. Hernandez, M. J., Brennan, R. W., and Bowman, G. S. Autoregulation of cerebral blood flow in the newborn dog. *Brain Res. 184*:199-202, 1980.
46. Pasternak, J. F., Groothuis, D. R., and Fisher, J. M. Regional variability of blood flow and glucose utilization within the subependymal germinal matrix. *Ann. Neurol. 12*:223, 1982.
47. Ashwal, S., Majcher, J. S., and Longo, L. D. Patterns of fetal lamb regional cerebral blood flow during and after prolonged hypoxia: studies during the posthypoxic recovery period. *Am. J. Ob Gyn. 139*:365-372, 1981.
48. Borgstrom, L., Johansson, II., and Siesju, B. K. The influence of acute normovolemic anemia on cerebral blood flow and oxygen consumption of anesthetized rats. *Acta. Physiol. Scand. 93*:505-514, 1975.
49. Johansson, H., and Siesjo, B. K. Cerebral blood flow and oxygen consumption in the rat in hypoxic hypoxia. *Acta Physiol. Scand. 93*:269-276, 1975.
50. Kety, S. S., and Schmidt, C. F. The effects of altered arterial tension of carbon dioxide and oxygen on cerebral blood flow and cerebral oxygen consumption of normal young men. *J. Clin. Invest. 27*:484, 1948.
51. Thomas, D. J., duBoulay, G. H., Marshall, J., et al. Effect of hematocrit on cerebral blood flow in man. *Lancet 2*:941-943, 1977.
52. Tweed, W. A., Cote, J., Wade, J. G., et al. Preservation of fetal brain blood flow relative to other organs during hypovolemic hypotension. *Pediatr. Res. 16*:137-140, 1982.
53. Sola, A., Spitzer, A. R., Morin, F. C., et al. Effects of arterial carbon dioxide tension on the newborn lamb's cardiovascular responses to rapid hemorrhage. *Pediatr. Res. 17*:70-76, 1983.
54. Laptook, A., Stonestreet, B. S., and Oh, W. The effects of different rates of plasmanate infusions upon brain blood flow after asphyxia and hypotension in newborn piglets. *J. Pediatr. 100*:791-796, 1982.
55. Laptook, A. R., Stonestreet, B. S., and Oh, W. Brain blood flow and O_2 delivery during hemorrhagic hypotension in the piglet. *Pediatr. Res. 17*:77-80, 1983.
56. Hernandez, M. J., Brennan, R. W., and Hawkins, R. A. Regional cerebral blood flow during neonatal asphyxia. In: *Cerebral Metabolism and Neural Function*, edited by J. V. Passonneau, R. A. Hawkins, W. D. Lust, and F. A. Welsh. Baltimore: Williams and Wilkins, 1980.
57. Bucciarelli, R. L., and Eitzman, D. V. Cerebral blood flow during acute acidosis in perinatal goats. *Pediart. Res. 13*:178-180, 1979.
58. Neligan, G. A., and Smith, C. A. The blood pressure of newborn infants in asphyxial states in hyaline membrane disease. *Pediatrics 26*:735-744, 1960.

59. Hill, A., Perlman, J. M., and Volpe, J. J. Relationship of pneumothorax to occurrence of intraventricular hemorrhage in the premature newborn. *Pediatrics 69*:144, 1982.
60. Vert, P., Nomin, P., and Sibout, M. Intracranial venous pressure in newborns: Variation in physiologic state and in neurologic and respiratory disorders. In: *Intensive Care in the Newborn*, edited by L. Stern. New York: Masson, 1975.
61. Bejar, R., Schneider, H., Osorno, L., et al. Association of early aortograms and PDA ligation with intraventricular hemorrhage (IVH). *Pediatr. Res. 15*: 650, 1981.
62. Marshall, T. A., Marshall, F., and Reddy, P. P. Physiologic changes associated with ligation of the ductus arteriosus in preterm infants. *J. Pediatr. 101*: 749-753, 1982.
63. Hill, A., Perlman, J. M., and Volpe, J. J. Identification of a syndrome with "steal" of blood from the cerebral arteries by left to right shunting of blood through a patent ductus arteriosus in premature infants. *Ann. Neurol. 10*: 301-302, 1981.
64. Bada, H. S., Hajjar, W., Chus, C., et al. Non-invasive diagnosis of neonatal asphyxia and intraventricular hemorrhage by Doppler ultrasound. *J. Pediatr. 95*:775-779, 1979.
65. Donn, S. M., Roloff, D. W., and Goldstein, G. W. Prevention of intraventricular haemorrhage in preterm infants by phenobarbitone. *Lancet 2*:215-217, 1981.
66. Morgan, M. E. I., Massey, R. F., and Cooke, R. W. I. Does phenobarbitone prevent periventricular hemorrhage in very low-birth-weight babies: a controlled trial. *Pediatrics 70*:186-189, 1982.
67. Wimberly, P. D., Lou, H. C., Pedersen, H., et al. Hypertensive peaks in the pathogenesis of intraventricular hemorrhage in the newborn. Abolition by phenobarbitone sedation. *Acta Paediatr. Scand. 71*:537-541, 1982.
68. Morgan, M. E. I., Benson, J. W. T., and Cooke, R. W. I. Ethamsylate reduces the incidence of periventricular haemorrhage in very low birthweight babies. *Lancet 2*:830-831, 1980.
69. Ment, L. R., Stewart, W. B., Scott, D. T., et al. Beagle puppy model of intraventricular hemorrhage: randomized indomethacin prevention trial. *J. Neurosurg. 58*:857-862, 1983.
70. Pickard, J. D., MacDonell, L. A., MacKenzie, E. T., et al. Response of the cerebral circulation in baboons to changing perfusion pressure after indomethacin. *Circ. Res. 40*:198-203, 1977.
71. Friedman, Z., and Berman, W. Hematologic effects of prostaglandins and thromboxanes and inhibitors of their synthesis in the perinatal period. In: *Prostaglandins in the Perinatal Period*, edited by M. A. Heymann. New York: Grune and Stratton, 1980.

CHAPTER 4

New Therapies for Asphyxia Neonatorum and Intraventricular Hemorrhage of the Premature

Gary W. Goldstein, M.D.

Recent advances in respiratory and cardiovascular support make it possible for many infants with severe asphyxia or intracranial hemorrhage to survive the neonatal period. It is the concern of all of us involved in the care of these infants that advanced skills in life support technology lead to the survival of children without neurological deficits. The goal of this review is to describe several new techniques to study the human nervous system and to indicate their potential role in the development of treatments to limit or reverse brain damage produced by asphyxia and hemorrhage.

The discovery of a method to image regional cerebral metabolism was one of the major breakthroughs in brain biochemistry during the past decade [1]. In this technique, radioactive analogues of glucose are used in conjunction with tissue autoradiography to determine the rate of glucose consumption in discrete regions of brain. In this way, enhanced regional metabolism is documented after activation of normal physiological events. For example, glucose consumption increases markedly in the occipital lobe following exposure of the eyes to light. Similarly, an increase in glucose metabolism occurs in the right frontal lobe, left cerebellar hemisphere, and anterior horn cells of the left side of the cervical spinal cord in association with movement of the left hand. This method to study regional brain

Perinatal Neurology and Neurosurgery. Edited by R. A. Thompson, J. R. Green, and S. D. Johnsen. Copyright © 1985 by Spectrum Publications, Inc.

metabolism was recently merged with computer-based tomography of the brain using isotopes of glucose-emitting positrons. Positron emission tomography (PET) allows the measurement of regional cerebral metabolism and its change during normal and abnormal brain activity in human subjects [2]. These studies should provide new information about the pathogenesis of brain tissue destruction after ischemia. Thus, changes in brain metabolism and circulation after primary insult may greatly enlarge the initial lesion and contribute more to the lasting neurological deficit than the original infarct.

Ten years ago with the advent of computerized tomography (CT) brain scans, it became possible to image brain anatomy and define the structural changes that occur after injury. This new radiologic technique also made it possible to determine the incidence of intracranial hemorrhage in premature infants [3]. For decades, it was assumed that such a hemorrhage was almost always fatal. We now know from information collected by performing CT brain scans on large populations of low-birthweight infants that the hemorrhages are usually not fatal and that as many as 40% of all small premature infants have this lesion. The extent of the hemorrhage appears to correlate with the degree of later neurological deficit. The most recent addition to imaging technology available to study this problem is the ultrasound scan. Using high resolution transducers, it is possible to image the intracranial contents through the anterior fontanel. The scans are simple to produce and require no sedation or restraint for the infant. The fact that ultrasound equipment is portable and does not use ionizing radiation permits frequent examinations to monitor the evolution of the hemorrhage. Using these imaging techniques, it has become clear that many premature infants with hemorrhage develop hydrocephalus days to weeks after the initial bleeding [4]. By combining serial ultrasound images with non-invasive measures of intracranial pressure, it is possible to evaluate therapy for the hydrocephalus. In our nursery, we institute a program of repeated lumbar punctures and begin to administer diuretics to infants with progressive ventriculomegaly. The therapy is begun prior to the development of increased intracranial pressure. We find that the hydrocephalus spontaneously remits in the majority of the infants managed in this fashion. Temporary or permanent ventricular diversions are performed in the few patients who do not respond to these conservative measures.

Radionuclear cisternal scans can be used to evaluate the integrity of spinal fluid pathways in premature infants with enlarged cerebral ventricles [5]. A radioactive tracer is placed within the lumbar spinal sac and images of the brain then document the diffusion of the tracer into the basilar cisterns. Early in the evolution of hydrocephalus, the isotope is unable to leave the cisterns and circulate over the convexity of the brain for absorption across the arachnoid villi into the sagital sinus. Instead, the isotope stagnates in the basilar cisterns and enters the ventricular cavities. When the hydrocephalus begins to resolve, isotope scans demonstrate a return to a normal flow of cerebrospinal fluid over the cerebral convexities and into venous blood. In most premature infants with posthemorrhagic hydrocephalus, this obstruction to the flow of cerebrospinal fluid is reversible with time. These results provide further evidence to support the initial use of conservative measures to manage posthemorrhagic hydrocephalus in premature infants [6].

Regional cerebral blood flow studies using the PET scan were recently performed on premature infants with periventricular hemorrhage to study changes in cerebral hemodynamics [7]. The first patients studied with this method had decreased blood flow in the regions surrounding the hemorrhage. The area of decreased blood flow was centered at the watershed and was much larger than the size of the hemorrhage defined by CT brain scan. The ischemia produced by this decrease in blood flow may be more damaging to the brain than the hemorrhage itself.

With ultrasound scans it is possible to closely monitor low-birthweight infants for the occurrence of intraventricular hemorrhage. This new imaging tool thus provides an excellent way to determine the effectiveness of measures to prevent these hemorrhages. Episodic abnormalities in cerebral blood flow have been proposed as a cause for hemorrhage in the premature baby [8]. In this model, surges in systemic blood pressure associated with a breakthrough in the normal autoregulatory mechanisms protecting the brain from hypertension cause an overperfusion of the capillary bed in the germinal matrix. Since the germinal matrix is undergoing involution during the third trimester of gestation, the tissue may be less supportive and make the capillaries more prone to rupture when they are overperfused with blood. Alternatively, this region may undergo ischemic infarction during episodes of hypotension because the matrix is in a watershed of the cerebral circulation. In fact, it is this exact watershed region of the matrix that is most likely to harbor a hemorrhage. Changes in blood pressure can be produced by noxious stimuli, hypoxia, or by a neurogenic mechanism. Seizures, for example, even when accompanied by only very minor motor phenomenon, produce marked increases in blood pressure and intracranial pressure [9].

Although not yet well defined, seizures in premature babies may also lead to redistribution of blood flow within the brain with diversion of flow to cortical areas of high metabolism associated with the seizure focus. Since it is at a watershed, the germinal matrix may become ischemic during activation of a seizure focus elsewhere in the brain. Repeated insults of this type may produce hemorrhage. With these possibilities in mind, investigations were started to test several drugs that might prevent or limit the size of cerebral hemorrhages in premature infants.

Phenobarbital was the first drug investigated as a preventive agent for intraventricular hemorrhage in premature infants [10]. It was administered in anticonvulsant dosages that should both provide protection from seizures as well as act as a mild sedative and a potential attenuator of blood pressure lability. The phenobarbital was given in a loading dose of 20 mg/kg body weight within the first hours of life to premature babies weighing less than 1500 gm. Infants were assigned to treatment or no-treatment groups by random lottery. Hemorrhage occurred in 15% of the treatment group which was significantly lower than the incidence of 42% in the control group. The survival rate was no different in the two groups. Since fewer survivors in the treatment group had hemorrhages, follow-up studies will be important to determine whether there is a difference in neurological outcome between these two groups. Another study using a different treatment protocol did not find a beneficial effect of phenobarbital upon the incidence of intraventricular hemorrhage in premature infants [11]. The conflicting results suggest that dose, timing of administration, and duration of therapy are important in determining effectiveness [12]. Several larger double-blind studies are now underway to further study the potential effectiveness of phenobarbital in this condition.

Ethamsylate is a drug capable of increasing the crosslinking between collagen molecules. In the hope of strengthening the blood vessel wall and other support tissues within the germinal matrix, this drug was administered to premature babies in an attempt to lower the incidence of hemorrhage [13]. Pretreatment produced a significant decrease in the incidence of hemorrhage from 51% in the control group to 26% on the treatment group. Ethamsylate also alters platelet adhesiveness and therefore has more than one potential mechanism of action in reducing intracranial hemorrhage.

The third drug study to prevent intracranial hemorrhage was performed in newborn puppies. Dogs are immature at birth and have a germinal matrix much like that of a human premature infant. By performing a delayed replacement exchange transfusion, it was possible to cause redistribution of blood volumes and blood pressure lability in the puppies. These hemodynamic changes resulted in a high rate of periventricular hemorrhages. To stabilize blood pressure during this stress and to change the pattern of blood vessel injury, newborn puppies were treated with indometheacin, an inhibitor of prostaglandin synthesis [14]. This drug decreased the blood pressure changes associated with the transfusion and greatly reduced the incidence of hemorrhage. The exact mechanism for reduction in hemorrhage in this experiment was unclear because prostaglandins are also involved in regulation of microvessel constriction and plate-let adhesiveness. Taken together, these pilot investigations are quite exciting in that they suggest that pharmacological intervention can reduce the incidence of intracranial hemorrhage in premature infants.

Recently, a great many investigations have been carried out on premature infants with intracranial hemorrhage. The interest was generated in part by the fact that these infants are treated in a limited number of tertiary care nurseries. In addition, the hemor-rhages are easy to visualize with modern scanning techniques. Even though these hemorrhages are common in low-birthweight infants, it should be remembered that the total number of term infants damaged by asphyxia greatly exceeds the number of preterm infants with intracranial hemorrhage. The impact of asphyxia neonatorum in terms of future cerebral palsy and mental retardation is therefore much greater than that of intracranial hemorrhage in the premature baby. Aside from obstetric measures to recognize asphyxia during labor and improve delivery techniques, little progress has been made to prevent the brain damage associated with this event. Diagnosis of asphyxia neonatorum is made by clinical evaluation rather than by brain imaging [15]. The severely asphyxiated infant has low Apgar scores, metabolic acidosis, and profound neurological depres-sion at birth. Convulsions are common but usually do not become clinically evident until the infant is between 12 and 24 hours of age. Once apparent, the convulsions are difficult to control and often require massive doses of medication. Brain edema producing increased intracranial pressure is also a common finding. The acute encephalopathy subsides after several days, but many babies are left with permanent neurological damage.

It will be important to determine whether events occurring after the initial resuscitation lead to further brain damage and whether pharmacological agents can prevent secondary extension of the injury. Disruption of the close regulation of cerebral blood flow to metabolic demand is one example of altered physiology that could lead to further brain damage. It is quite possible that the metabolic demands of the recurrent convulsions are not met by adequate circulatory responses and that further injuries to the brain occur during the several days of seizure activity. A multi-institution trial of anticonvulsant medications given prior to onset of the seizures in infants with clinical signs of severe asphyxia is now in the planning stages. This study is based on the hypothesis that preventing convulsions during the second and third day of life will decrease permanent neurological deficits.

During the past several years, there has been a growing interest in brain endorphins and their role in normal and abnormal brain responses. These peptides are the endogenous opiates of the brain. They may normally modulate response to pain and appear to be released after brain injury. It is possible that these natural opiate-like molecules are involved in the neurological depression associated with severe asphyxia neonatorum. If endorphins are released in large quantities after asphyxia, they may not only depress respiration and alertness but interfere with normal regulation of cerebral blood flow. Naloxone is a potent pharmacological inhibitor of opiate action. Experiments with newborn animals suggest that naloxone reduces the neurological depression associated with asphyxia [16]. If this were true in humans, the drug might prove useful in the treatment of asphyxia during the initial resuscitation. In addition to depression, release of endorphins may cause abnormalities in the function of the microcirculation after the anoxic injury. This potential pathogenic role of peptides has been best studied in animals with spinal cord injury. In this experimental setting, both naloxone [17] and thyrotropin-releasing hormone, a natural biologic inhibitor of opiates, were found effective in limiting the extent of damage following traumatic injury [19]. These studies suggest that pharmacological intervention after the occurrence of an insult to the nervous system might limit the extent of injury and improve ultimate outcome.

A final class of new pharmacological agents, the calcium blockers, may also prove to have a role in treating brain injuries in the neonate. Abnormal entry of calcium into a cell appears to be a final common mechanism of cell injury and death [19]. Under normal circumstances the concentration of ionized calcium inside a cell is 10,000-fold lower than the concentration of ionized calcium in the extracellular fluid. This difference in concentration is maintained by energy-dependent pumps that actively transport calcium from the inside of the cell to the outside. In addition, the plasma membrane of a normal cell is usually impermeable to calcium ions. In normal cells, the internal concentration of calcium is closely regulated and serves to control the activities of several intracellular enzymes and contractile elements. Thus, stimulation of smooth muscle cells leads to an enhanced permeability of calcium channels in the plasma membrane. Calcium ions enter the cell and cause the muscle fibers to contract. When a cell is damaged, the plasma membrane becomes more permeable to calcium. If energy stores are depleted and other ion gradients are dissipated, it will be difficult to pump the calcium out of the cell. In this circumstance, calcium accumulates in the mitochondria and this further limits energy production. The end result can be cell death and pathological calcifications. When this occurs in the smooth muscle cells of a blood vessel, abnormal constrictions will occur due to pathological activation of contractile elements within the vessel wall. Not only will the cells of the blood vessel be damaged, but the abnormal constriction can produce inadequate blood flow to the brain. In this way an ischemic event may begin a cascade of events leading to a progressive increase in the size of the brain lesion. The ability to limit the abnormal entry of calcium into an injured cell might avert some steps in this damaging cycle. The calcium-blocking agents offer the potential for such a pharmacological intervention [20]. The use of these drugs is best studied in cardiovascular disorders. However, several of the newer calcium-blocking agents are able to enter the brain and alter cerebral blood flow. A recent study of patients with subarachnoid hemorrhage suggests that calcium blockers may be useful in preventing the blood vessel spasm that commonly occurs after brain hemorrhage [21].

The next decade looks promising for learning more about the pathogenesis of brain injuries in the newborn and developing a rational program of pharmacological interventions. The new imaging techniques will allow us to visualize the structural and metabolic responses to injury. With new pharmacological agents and a better understanding of brain metabolism we should be able to improve the neurological outcome of sick newborn infants.

REFERENCES

1. Sokoloff, L. Localization of functional activity in the central nervous system by measurement of glucose utilization with radioactive deoxyglucose. *J. Cereb. Blood Flow Metabol.* 1:7-36, 1981.

2. Phelps, M. E., Mazziotta, J. C., and Huang, S.-C. Study of cerebral function with positron computed tomography. *J. Cereb. Blood Flow Metabol. 2*: 113-162, 1982.
3. Papile, L. A., Burstein, J., Burstein, R., et al. Incidence and evolution of subependymal and intraventricular hemorrhage: A study of infants with birth weights less than 1,500 gm. *J. Pediatrics 92*:529, 1978.
4. Donn, S. M., Goldstein, G. W., and Silver, T. M. Real-time ultrasonography: Its use in the evaluation of neonatal intracranial hemorrhage and post-hemorrhagic hydrocephalus. *Am. J. Dis. Child. 135*:319, 1981.
5. Donn, S. M., Roloff, D. W., and Keyes, J. W., Jr. Evaluation of neonatal hydrocephalus by radionuclide lumbar cisternography. *Pediatrics*, in press, 1983.
6. Goldstein, G. W., Chaplin, E. R., and Maitland, J. Transient hydrocephalus in premature infants: Treatment by lumbar punctures. *Lancet i*:512, 1976.
7. Volpe, J. J., Perlman, J. M., Herscovitch, P. et al. Positron emission tomography in the assessment of regional cerebral blood flow in the newborn. *Ann. Neurol. 12*:225, 1982.
8. Wimberley, P. D., Lou, H. C., Pedersen, H., et al. Hypertensive peaks in the pathogenesis of intra-ventricular hemorrhage in the newborn: Abolition by phenobarbitone sedation. *Acta. Paediatr. Scand. 71*:537-542, 1982.
9. Perlman, J. M., and Volpe, J. J. Seizures in the preterm infant: Effects on cerebral blood flow metabolism, intracranial pressure, and arterial blood pressure. *J. Pediatrics 102*:288-293, 1983.
10. Donn, S. M., Roloff, D. W., and Goldstein, G. W. Prevention of intracranial haemorrhage in preterm infants by phenobarbitone. *Lancet 2*:215-217, 1981.
11. Morgan, M. E. I., Massey, R. F., and Cooke, R. W. I. Does phenobarbitone prevent periventricular hemorrhage in very low-birth-weight babies?: A controlled trial. *Pediatrics 70*:186-189, 1982.
12. Goldstein, G. W., Donn, S. M., and Roloff, D. W. Further observations on the use of phenobarbital to prevent neonatal intracranial hemorrhage. *Pediatrics 70*:1014-1015, 1982.
13. Morgan, M. E. I., Benson, J. W. T., and Cooke, R. W. I. Ethamsylate reduces the incidence of periventricular haemorrhage in very low-birth-weight babies. *Lancet ii*:830-831, 1981.
14. Ment, L. R., Stewart, W. B., Scott, D. T., and Duncan, C. C. Beagle puppy model of intraventricular hemorrhage: Randomized indomethacin prevention trial. *Neurology 33*:179-184, 1983.
15. Brown, J. K., Purvis, R. J., Forfar, J. O., and Cockburn, F. Neurological aspects of perinatal asphyxia. *Dev. Med. Child. Neurol. 16*:567-580, 1974.
16. Chernick, V. and Craig, R. J. Naloxone reserves neonatal depression caused by fetal asphyxia. *Science 216*:1252-1253, 1982.
17. Faden, A. I., Jacobs, T. P., and Holaday, J. W. Opiate antagonist improves neurologic recovery after spinal injury. *Science 211*:493-494, 1981.
18. Faden, A. I., Jacobs, T. P., and Holaday, J. W. Thyrotropin-releasing hormone improves neurologic recovery after spinal trauma in cats. *N. Engl. J. Med. 305*:1063-1067, 1981.
19. Godfraind, T. Mechanisms of action of calcium entry blockers. *Federation Proc. 40*:2866-2871, 1981.

20. Harris, R. J., Branston, N. M., Symon, L., et al. The effects of a calcium antagonist, Nimodipine, upon physiological response of the cerebral vasculature and its possible influence upon focal cerebral ischemia. *Stroke 13*: 759-766, 1982.
21. Allen, G. S., Ahn, H. S., Preziosi, T. J., et al. Cerebral arterial spasm— A controlling trial of Nimodipine in patients with subarachnoid hemorrhage. *N. Engl. J. Med. 308*:619-624, 1983.

CHAPTER 5

Cranial Sonography and CT of the Infant

Diane S. Babcock, M.D.

INDICATIONS

Improvements in neonatal care in the past few years have resulted in fewer respiratory deaths, and neurological problems have become the limiting factor in neonatal prognosis. Both CT and ultrasound are useful for evaluating the newborn brain. The indications for brain scanning include (1) screening for brain anomalies in patients with other anomalies such as meningomyelocele and midline facial cleft defects; (2) screening for, and follow-up of, intracranial hemorrhage; (3) unexplained seizures; (4) enlarged head by measurement; (5) trauma; (6) increased intracranial pressure; (7) meningitis not responding to therapy; (8) intrauterine infections; (9) abnormal neurological examinations; (10) suspected malfunction of ventricular shunt; (11) intraoperative positioning of shunt catheter; and (12) birth asphyxia.

Certain lesions will be better evaluated by one modality or the other, but many can be equally well evaluated with either. When the expected abnormality can be evaluated with either modality, ultrasound would generally be the method of choice because it is portable, less expensive, and uses no ionizing radiation. CT is reserved for those situations where ultrasonography does not adequately image the area—such as subdural hematomas and hygromas in trauma and meningitis and, when further evaluation is necessary, such as complex congenital anomalies, tumors, anoxic brain damage

Perinatal Neurology and Neurosurgery. Edited by R. A. Thompson, J. R. Green, and S. D. Johnsen. Copyright © 1985 by Spectrum Publications, Inc.

in full-term infants, and seizure patients with normal ultrasound examinations.

TECHNIQUE—ULTRASOUND

The examinations are performed portably in the newborn intensive care unit with a real-time machine when the baby is unstable or on a respirator. When the infant is stable enough to be moved, the examinations are performed in the radiology department using contact (Figure 1) and real-time scanners. Sedation is not usually necessary, although chloral hydrate in an oral dose of 50 mg/kg may be given on follow-up examinations and in older infants. Warmed aqueous gel is placed on the infant's head as a couplant. Five to seven MHz transducers are used for newborns and three to five MHz transducers for older infants. Serial scans of the head are performed in coronal and sagittal planes in five mm intervals with a real-time scanner. Coronal and axial series are performed with a contact scanner when the patient is examined in the radiology department. Information is obtained by scanning through the open sutures and

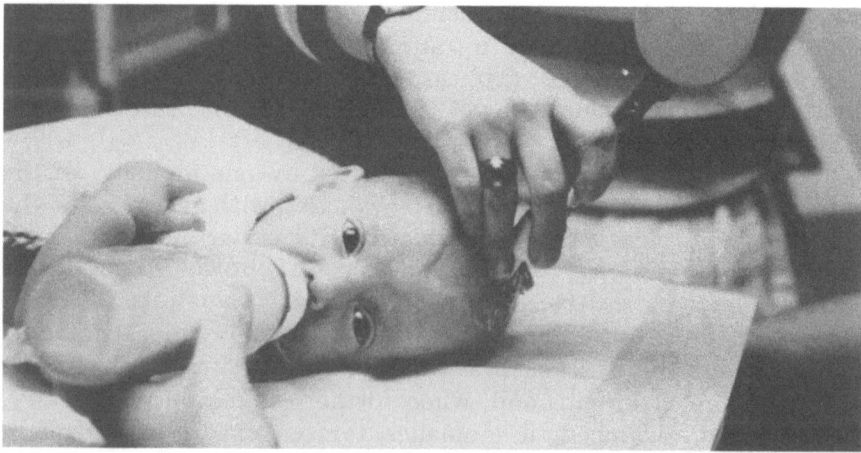

Figure 1. Sonographer performing ultrasound scan of head through anterior fontanel in coronal plane. (Reproduced with permission from Babcock D. S. and Han, B. K. *Cranial Ultrasonography of Infants.* Baltimore: Williams and Wilkins, 1981).

fontanels, so only children under two years of age can be examined with this technique.

The advantages of real-time include: portability, speed, lower cost, and less technical experience and ability are required. Limitations of real-time scanners include: near-field artifact obliterates small amounts of fluid in interhemispheric fissure, incomplete sector of the head, resolution possible is less than with contact scanners. Sector scanners are preferable to linear arrays because of poor contact with head.

TECHNIQUE—CT

Sedation is necessary in occasional patients, particulary those given intravenous contrast material. The I.V. is started in a peripheral vein prior to examination and the infant is monitored and observed by a radiology department nurse throughout the exam. The temperature in the scanning room is kept at 75 to 80 degrees and even higher when preterm infants are examined. Radiant heaters can also be used to warm the infant. The infant's arms and legs are restrained with Velcro straps, wristlets, and sandbags. The head position is maintained with a head-holder (Figure 2). Providing a darkened, warm,

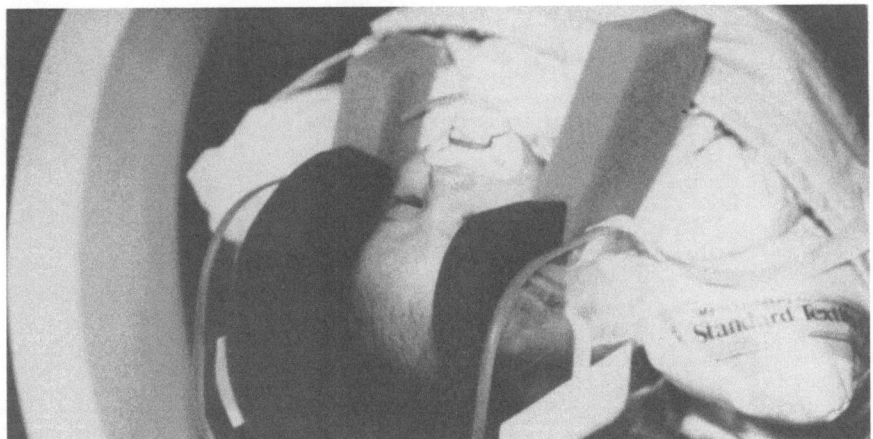

Figure 2. Infant's head position maintained in CT gantry with head-holder. (Modified from Derek Harwood-Nash, M.D., Toronto, Ontario.)

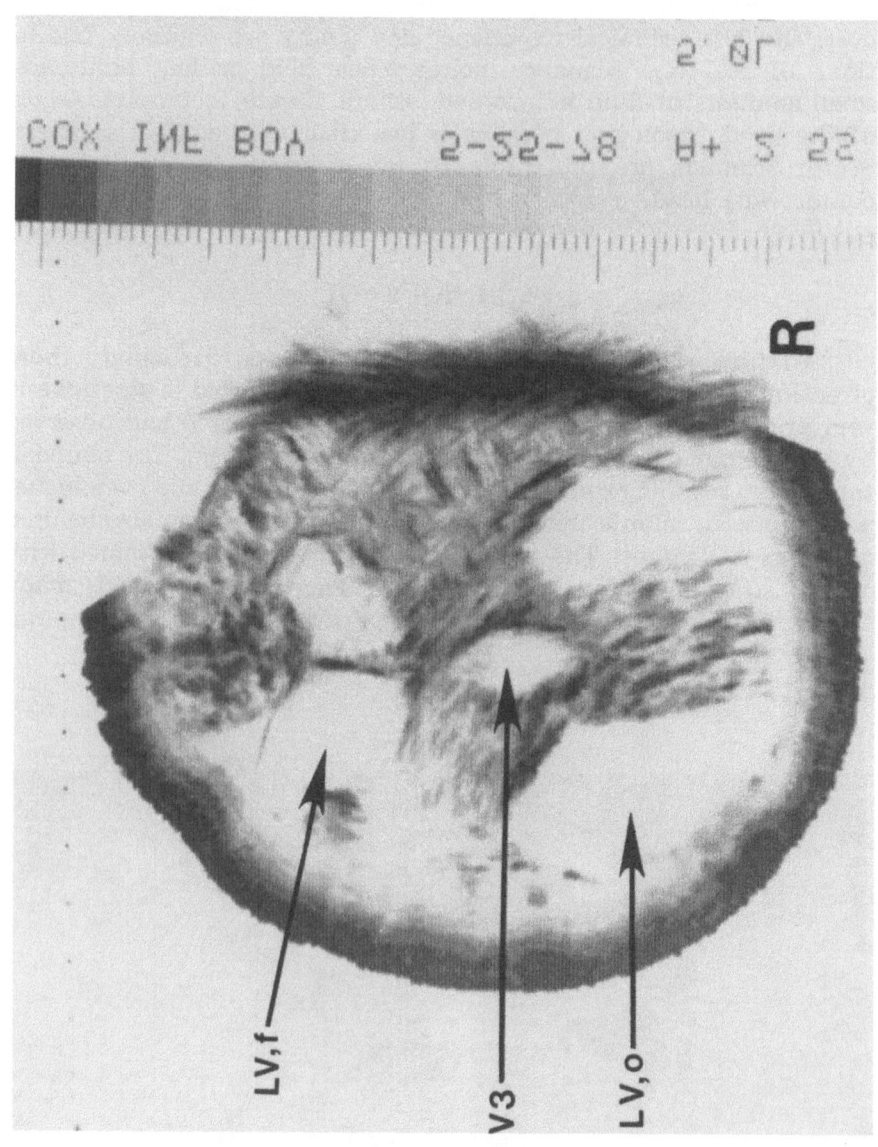

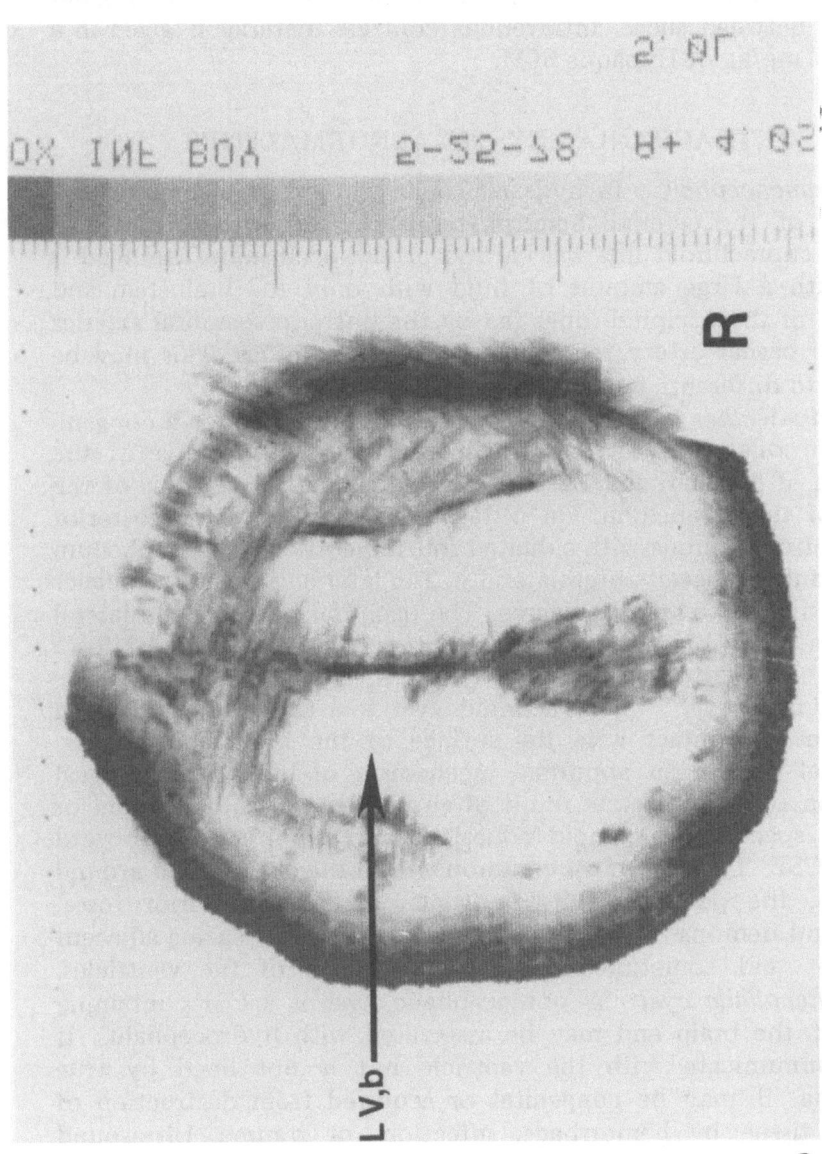

Figure 3. Hydrocephalus in seven-day-old infant with lumbosacral meningomyelocele and large head. (a, b), Axial scans. Moderate dilatation of frontal horns (LV,f), bodies (LV,b), and occipital horns (LV,o) of lateral ventricles and third ventricle (V3). Thickness of moderately echogenic cerebral cortex can be measured. (Reproduced with permission from Babcock D. S., Han B. K., and LeQuesne G. W. B-Mode gray scale ultrasound of the head in the newborn and young infant. *A. J. R. 134*: 457–468, 1980.)

and quiet environment and stroking the infant are helpful. An effort is made to speak in a soothing tone, distinctly but softly. Scans are performed in the dynamic scanning mode with short but regular intervals between slices. Intravenous contrast material is given in a dose of 2 mg/kg of Hypaque 60M.

INTRACRANIAL CYSTIC ABNORMALITIES

Hydranencephaly. In hydranencephaly, there is a massive destruction of the cerebral hemispheres associated with intrauterine bilateral supraclinoid internal carotid artery occlusion. The head is filled with a large amount of fluid with only the brainstem and portions of the occipital lobes fed by the posterior cerebral arteries from the basilar artery remaining. The falx is intact. This may be difficult to differentiate from severe hydrocephalus.

Dandy-Walker cyst. The Dandy-Walker syndrome is a congenital cystic dilatation of the fourth ventricle with atresia of the foramina of Magendi and Luschka associated with dysgenesis of the vermis of the cerebellum. On ultrasound, there is a large posterior fossa cyst continuous with a dilated fourth ventricle. The cerebellum is small and displaced anterolaterally. The lateral and third ventricles may be dilated to varying degree. The occipital horns of the lateral ventricles are displaced upwards and laterally by the posterior fossa cyst and elevated tentorium.

Arachnoid cyst. The arachnoid cyst is a CSF fluid collection which lies in contact with the surface of the brain and may be congenital due to an abnormal mechanism of the leptomeningeal formation or acquired as a result of entrapment of subarachnoid or cisternal space by arachnoid adhesions and unidirectional inward flow of CSF. They are most common within the cisterns and around the sella, the posterior third ventricle, and the posterior fossa. Ultrasound demonstrates a fluid containing space displacing adjacent structures and sometimes causing obstruction of the ventricles.

Porencephalic cyst. A porencephalic cyst is a CSF-containing cavity of the brain and may be associated with hydrocephalus. It may communicate with the ventricle but is not lined by true ependyma. It may be congenital or acquired from destruction of cerebral tissue by hemorrhage, infection, or trauma. Ultrasound demonstrates a fluid-containing mass communicating with the ventricle.

Congenital hydrocephalus. (Figure 3): Hydrocephalus may occur *in utero* due to a variety of etiologies. Ultrasonography will demonstrate dilatation of the ventricles proximal to the level of obstruction. Aqueductal stenosis, either primary or secondary to the Chiari II malformation, is probably the most common.

NONCYSTIC MALFORMATIONS OF THE BRAIN

Chiari II (Arnold-Chiari) malformation. The Chiari II malformation includes elongation of the pons and fourth ventricle and downward displacement of the medulla and fourth ventricle into the cervical spinal canal with a relatively small posterior fossa. The tectum is beaked and hydrocephalus of varying degree occurs due to aqueductal stenosis. This malformation is always associated with some form of spinal dysraphism, usually a meningomyelocele. Ultrasound demonstrates hydrocephalus which may be mild to marked and may be asymmetric. The lateral ventricles are characteristically pointed anteriorly with a medial concavity of the frontal horns. There is inferior pointing of the frontal horns resulting from prominence of the caudate nuclei. The septum pellucidum is frequently absent. The third ventricle frequently has an enlarged massa intermedia and a prominent anterior commissure. The posterior fossa is relatively small with a low lying tentorium. The tentorial-cerebellar pseudomass can be seen on low axial scans. The interhemispheric fissure is frequently prominent.

Agenesis of the corpus callosum. The corpus callosum is the principle tract connecting the right and left cerebral hemispheres and may be partially or completely absent. It normally forms the roof of the lateral ventricles. Ultrasound demonstrates separation of the lateral ventricles with increased angulation of the roofs in the region of the frontal horns and bodies. The third ventricle is dilated and herniates superiorly between the lateral ventricles. The septum pellucidum is absent. Hydrocephalus may occur secondary to an associated malformation such as aqueductal stenosis.

Holoprosencephaly. Holoprosencephaly results from a disorder of diverticulation of the fetal brain with a defect in midline cleavage of the prosencephalon which causes failure of formation of the separate cerebral hemispheres. This may be of varying severity and is often associated with midline facial malformations. The most severe form—alobar holoprosencephaly—demonstrates a small amount of cerebral tissue peripherally and anteriorly with no division into cerebral hemispheres. There is a large horseshoe-shaped single ventricular cavity and frequently fusion of the thalami. Lobar and

semilobar holoprosencephaly have partial separation into cerebral
hemispheres of varying degree; however, the frontal lobes are always
fused and the cerebral sagittal falx is only partially developed.

Arteriovenous malformations. Arteriovenous malformations of
the brain may occur in any location, but the Galenic malformation
(vein of Galen aneurysm) is the most common. Ultrasound demonstrates a mass displacing the normal structures which may be sonolucent due to liquid blood within the aneurysm or may be echogenic
due to thrombosed blood. Dilated ventricles may be present due to
obstruction by the mass or a previous subarachnoid hemorrhage.
Pulsation of the mass or surrounding dilated feeding vessels can be
identified with real-time sonography. Doppler demonstrates flow
within the malformation.

Tuberous sclerosis. Tuberous sclerosis is a histogenic malformation with hamartomas of fibrocellular nature involving many areas of
the body. In the brain there are subependymal and cortical tubers
and calcifications that can be detected as echogenic periventricular
or subependymal masses on ultrasonography.

INTRACRANIAL TUMORS

Tumors are relatively rare in this age group but do occur. They
can be identified on ultrasound by their abnormal echogenicity—
usually greater than that of normal brain, mass effect, and obstruction of the ventricles. CT and angiography are usually necessary
for complete evaluation; however, tumors are occasionally encountered when scanning patients for other problems.

INFECTIOUS DISEASES

Ultrasound is performed in patients with meningitis, not responding adequately to therapy, to look for subdural effusions and
empyemas and brain abscesses. CT is performed in those patients
when a small fontanel precludes adequate evaluation of the subdural
space and when an abnormality is strongly suspected clinically but
ultrasound is negative.

CRANIAL HEMORRHAGE

Cephalohematoma. The hematoma can be seen separating the
skin from the bony calvarium and may be sonolucent or have low

level echoes within it. Underlying fractures and subdural hematoma should be looked for. Reverberation artifacts cause problems if one scans over the cephalohematoma, so the head should be scanned from the opposite side.

Subdural hematomas. These hematomas are seen as a separation of the brain from the bony calvarium by sonolucent fluid. Small amounts of extra-axial fluid are best seen in the interhemispheric fissure under the fontanel. Subdural hematomas may be easily missed when small or localized over the convexities because of problems imaging this area, particularly in patients with small fontanels. CT is considered more accurate in these patients.

Intracerebral hemorrhage in full-term infants. This hemorrhage is usually due to birth trauma and is most common in the frontal and parietal regions. Acute hemorrhage is seen as an echogenic mass which gradually liquifies and frequently results in an area of porencephaly. There may be associated hydrocephalus due to obstruction of the CSF pathways by clot or arachnoiditis.

Intracranial hemorrhage in premature infants. This hemorrhage originates in the subependymal germinal matrix, which is largest in the 24 to 32 week-gestational infant. The incidence is reported at about 40 to 60% in infants under 32-week gestation. The germinal matrix is most prominent in the region of the caudothalamic groove in the inferolateral wall of the lateral ventricle. Subependymal hemorrhage is seen as increased echoes in the region of the caudate nucleus, most frequently the head. This may gradually resolve or result in a subependymal cyst.

Intraventricular hemorrhage occurs usually from rupture of the subependymal hemorrhage into the ventricle, but also may originate from a choroid plexus hemorrhage. This is diagnosed by echogenic clot or clot fluid level in the ventricle (Figure 4). Hydrocephalus may result from obstruction of the CSF pathways by clot or arachnoiditis and may be communicating or noncommunicating.

Intraparenchymal hemorrhage occurs by extension of the subependymal hemorrhage into the adjacent brain parenchyma or as a hemorrhagic infarct in the periventricular white matter. Hemorrhage is seen as a diffuse area of increased echoes extending in the brain parenchyma (Figure 5). Porencephaly results when an intraparenchymal hemorrhage undergoes liquefaction and cavitation of the involved brain.

It is currently recommended from data collected recently that all patients under 32-week gestation or 1500 gm be routinely screened by ultrasound at days 4 to 7 and at day 14 for ICH and ventricular

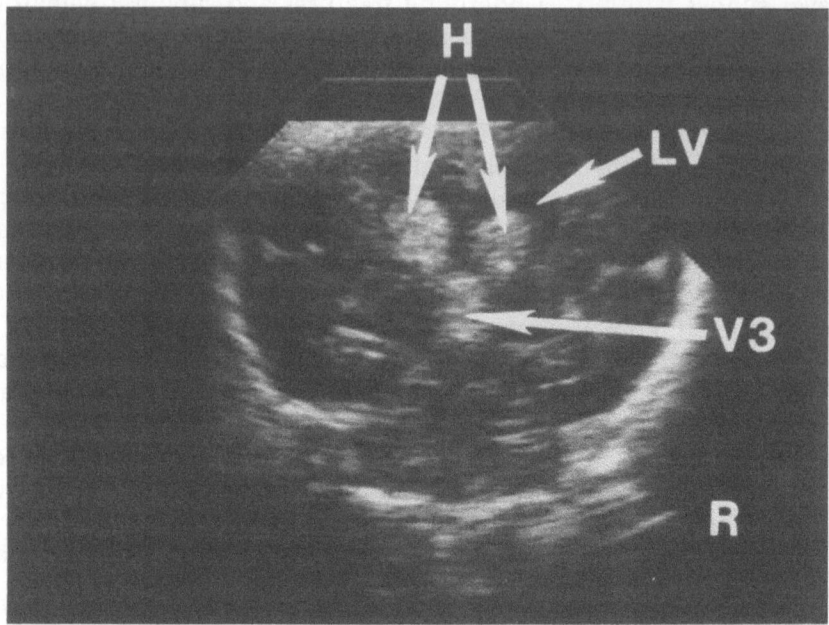

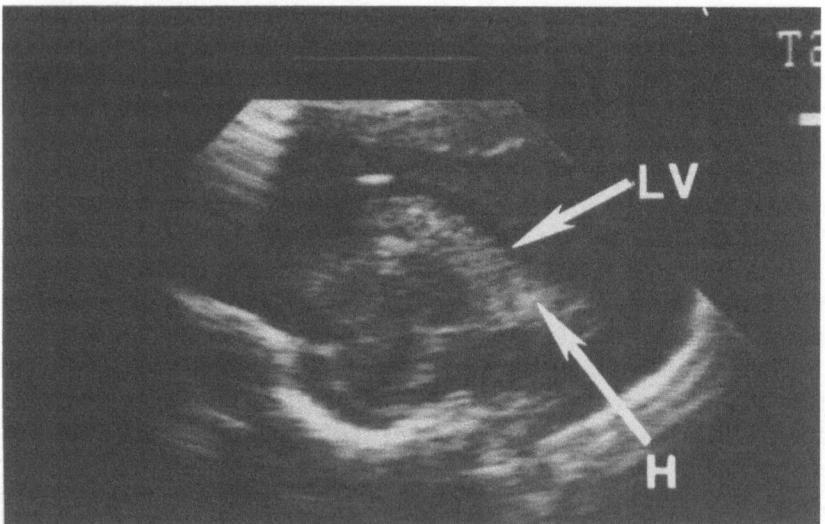

Figure 4. Intraventricular hemorrhage and hydrocephalus in 32-week gestation infant. Coronal (a) and parasagittal (b) sonograms on day 4 of life demonstrate bilateral hemorrhage (H) in region of caudate nucleus and within dilated lateral (LV) and third ventricles (V3). Coronal (c) and parasagittal (d) sonograms 2 weeks later demonstrate moderately dilated ventricles with liquifying blood

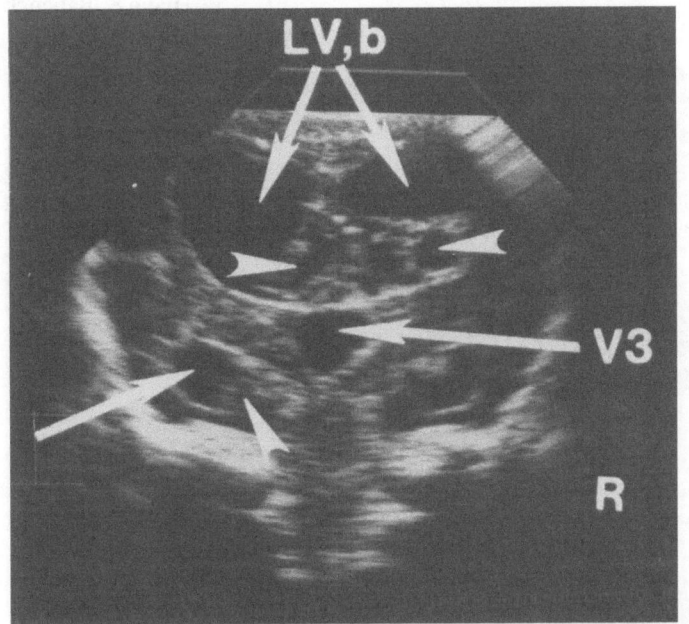

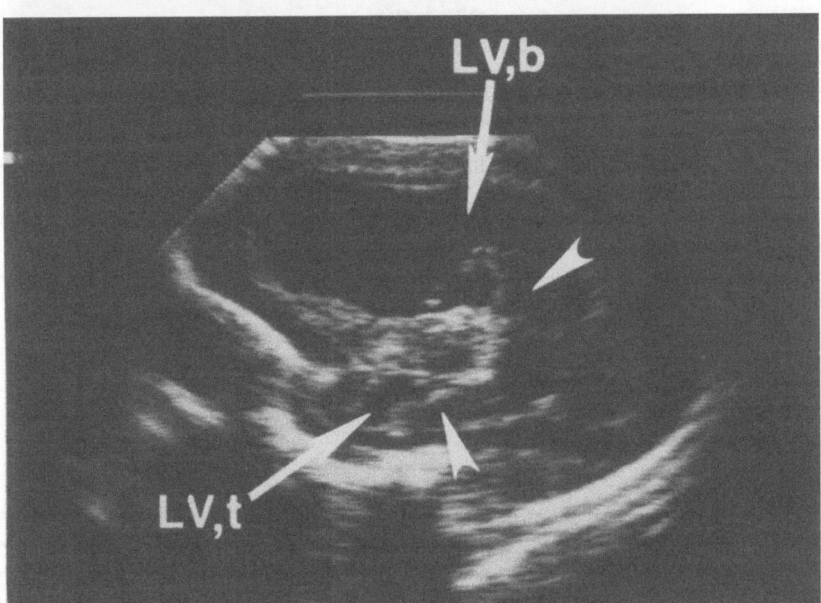

clots (arrowhead). LV,b = body of lateral ventricles; LV,t = temporal horn of lateral ventricles. (Reproduced with permission from Babcock D. S., Bove K. E., and Han B. K. Intracranial hemorrhage in premature infants: Sonographic-pathologic correlation. *A.J.N.R.* *3*:309–317, 1982.)

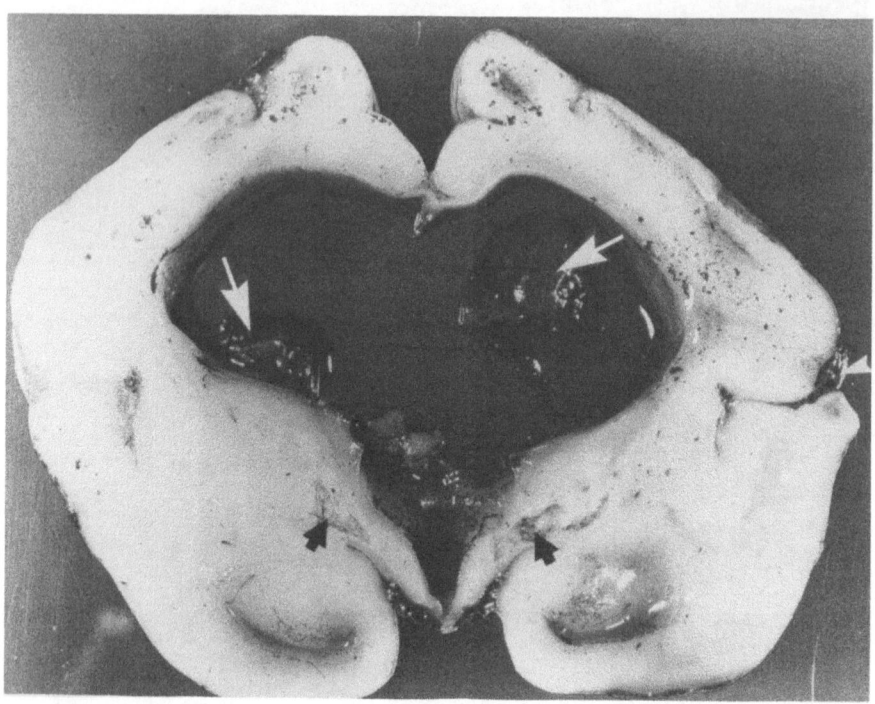

Figure 4. (e) Brain section same day as last sonogram shows moderate hydro-cephalus with blood clots in lateral ventricles (white arrows) and old subarach-noid hemorrhage (curved arrows). Bilateral infarction in globus pallidus (black arrows). (Reproduced with permission from Babcock D. S., Bove K. E., and Han B. K. Intracranial hemorrhage in premature infants: Sonographic-pathologic correlation. *A.J.N.R.* *3*:309–317, 1982.)

Figure 5. Intraparenchymal hemorrhage in 28-week gestation infant. A, Coronal sonogram demonstrates echogenic hemorrhage extending into peri-ventricular brain parenchyma. Right lateral ventricle and third ventricle (V3) filled with echogenic clot. Left lateral ventricle (LV) moderately enlarged. B, Brain section 9 days later shows bilateral subepenymal hemorrhage, asym-metrical intraventricular hemorrhage, and multiple foci of intraparenchymal extension (arrowheads). (Reproduced with permission from Babcock D. S., Bove K. E., and Han B. K. Intracranial hemorrhage in premature infants: Sonographic-pathologic correlation. *A.J.N.R.* *3*:309–317, 1982.)

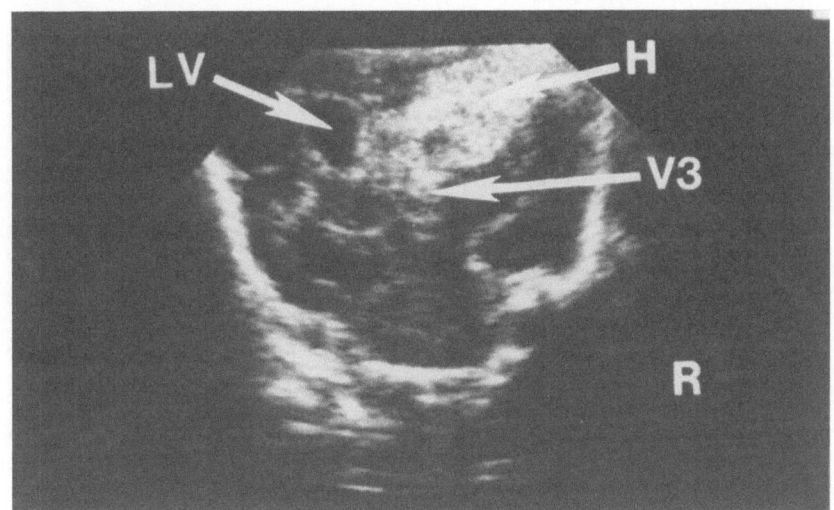

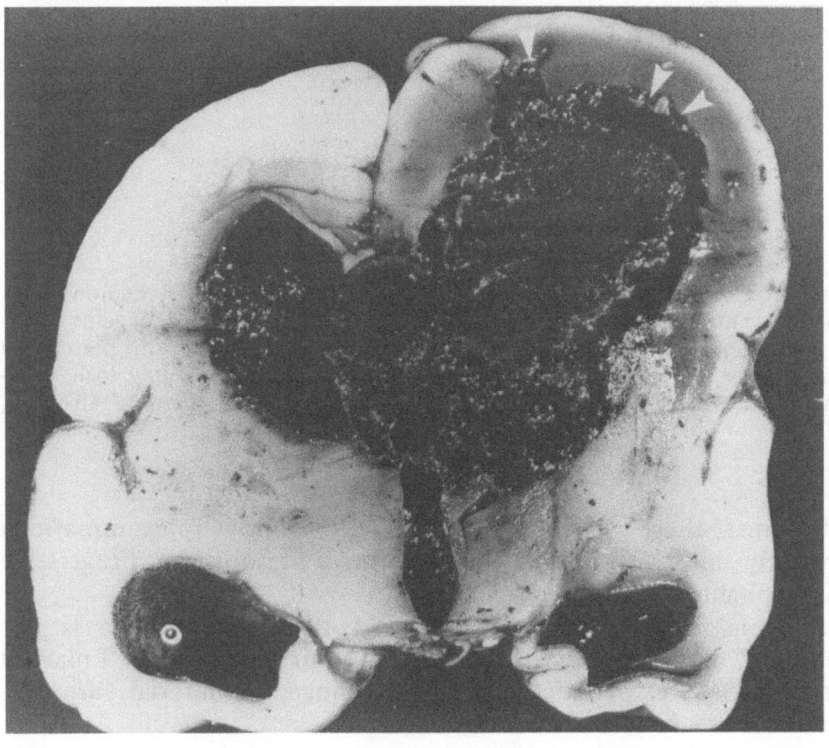

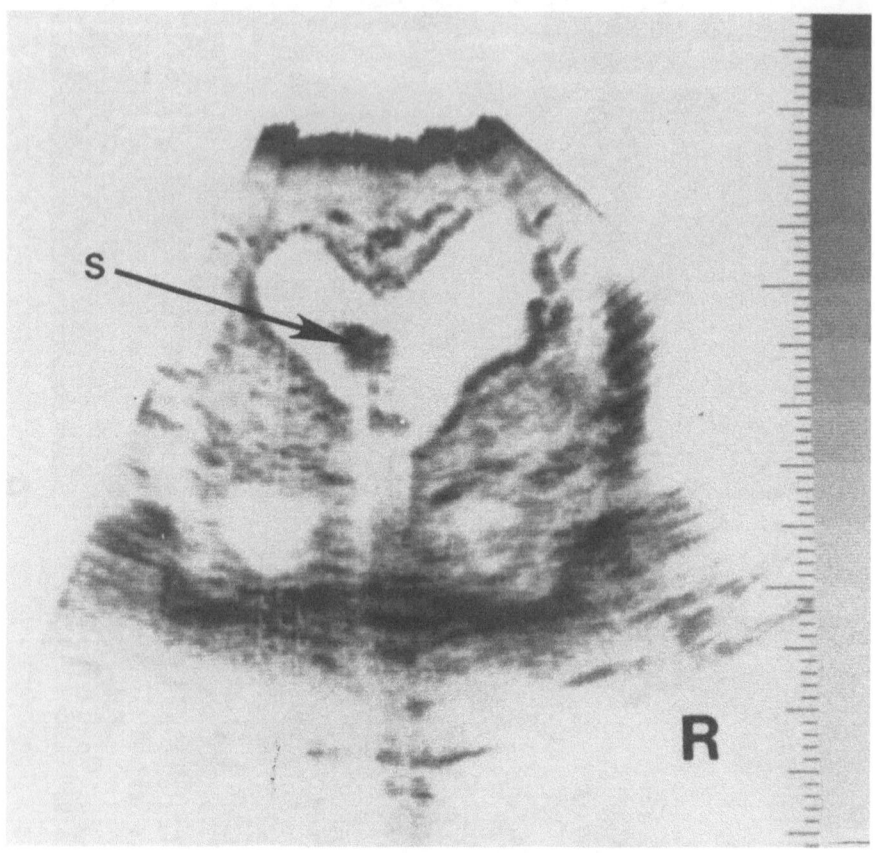

Figure 6. Coronal ultrasound scan after patient was shunted demonstrates moderate ventricular dilation with shunt catheter, (S) seen as echogenic structure with acoustical shadowing in the ventricle. (Reproduced with permission from Babcock D. S., Han B. K., and LeQuesne G. W. B-Mode gray scale ultrasound of the head in the newborn and young infant. *A.J.R. 134*:457–468, 1980.)

dilatation. If these scans are abnormal, then follow-up examinations at weekly intervals should be performed to look for progressive hydrocephalus.

Subarachnoid hemorrhage. This type of hemorrhage is not accurately diagnosed by ultrasound in our experience. Enlarged extra-axial spaces, particularly with echogenic material, are suspicious for arachnoid hemorrhage.

Cerebellar hemorrhage. This hemorrhage is relatively uncommon, but occurs particularly in full-term infants. Increased
echoes are seen in the cerebellum on ultrasound.

INTRAOPERATIVE USES OF ULTRASOUND

Ultrasound can be used in the operating room to visualize the
position of the shunt catheter as it is placed into the lateral ventricle,
usually the frontal horn (Figure 6). It can also be used intraopera-
tively to assist in the drainage of fluid collections and for localization for biopsy of deep tumors.

ADVANTAGES OF ULTRASONOGRAPHY FOR EXAMINING
THE INFANT HEAD

1. Nonionizing radiation
2. Brain can be imaged in multiple planes
3. Lower in cost
4. No sedation necessary in most infants
5. Noninvasive
6. Portable

REFERENCES

1. Babcock D. S., Han B. K., *Cranial Ultrasonography in Infants.* Baltimore:
   Williams and Wilkins, 1981.
2. Babcock D. S., Han B. K. Cranial sonographic findings in meningomyelocele. *A.J.N.R. 1*:493–499, 1980.
3. Babcock D. S., Han B. K., and LeQuesne G. W. B-mode gray scale ultrasound of the head in the newborn and young infant. *A.J.R. 134*:457–468,
   1980.
4. Babcock D. S., and Han B. K. The accuracy of high resolution, real-time
   ultrasonography of the head in infancy. *Radiology 139*:665–676, 1981.
5. Babcock D. S., Bove K., and Han B. K. Intracranial hemorrhage in premature infants: sonographic-pathologic correlation. *A.J.N.R. 3*:309–317,
   1982.
6. Chaplin E. R., et al. Posthemorrhagic hydrocephalus in the preterm infant.
   Pediatrics 65:901, 1981.
7. Cubberley D. A., Jaffe R. B., and Nixon G. W. Sonographic demonstration
   of galenic arteriovenous malformations in the neonate. *A.J.N.R. 3*:435–
   439, 1982.

8. Enzmann D. R., et al. The natural history of experimental intracerebral hemorrhage: sonography, computed tomography, and neuropathology. *A.J.N.R. 2*:517–526, 1981.

9. Farruggia S., and Babcock D. S. The cavum septi pellucidi: its appearance and incidence with cranial ultrasonography in infancy. *Radiology 139*: 147–150, 1981.

10. Fitzhardinge P. M., Flodmark O., Fitz C. R., and Ashby B. A. The prognostic value of computed tomography as an adjunct to assessment of the term infant with postasphyxial encephalopathy. *J. Pediatr. 99*:777–781, 1981.

11. Fleischer A. C., et al. Cranial sonography of the preterm neonate. *Diagnostic Imaging*, 1981.

12. Grant E. G., et al. Real-time ultrasonography of neonatal intraventricular hemorrhage and comparison with computed tomography. *Radiology 139*: 687–691, 1981.

13. Grant E. G., et al. Evolution of porencephalic cysts from intraparenchymal hemorrhage in neonates: sonographic evidence. *A.J.N. 3*:47, 1982.

14. Haber K., Wachter R. D., Christenson P. C., Yaucher Y., Sahn D. J., and Smith J. R. Ultrasonic evaluation of intracranial pathology in infants: a new technique. *Radiology 134*:173–178, 1980.

15. Hadlock F. P., Garcia-Prats J. A., Courtney J. T., and Park S. K. Sonographic diagnosis of neonatal intracranial hemorrhage. *Perinatology-Neonatology*, 1983.

16. Harwood-Nash D. C., and Fitz C. R. *Neuroradiology in Infants and Children.* St. Louis: C. V. Mosby, 1976.

17. Harwood-Nash D. C., et al. Diagnostic imaging of the neonatal brain: review and protocol. *A.J.N.R. 3*:103–115, 1982.

18. Hill A., Melson L., Clark B. H., et al. Hemorrhagic periventricular leukomalacia: diagnosis by real time ultrasound and correlation with autopsy findings. *Pediatrics 69*:282–284, 1982.

19. Hobar J. D., et al. Ultrasound detection of changing ventricular size in posthemorrhagic hydrocephalus. *Pediatrics 66*:674–678, 1980.

20. Johnson M. L., et al. Detection of neonatal intracranial hemorrhage utilizing real-time and static ultrasound. *Clin. Ultrasound 9*:427–433, 1981.

21. Johnson M. L., and Rumack C. M. Ultrasonic evaluation of the neonatal brain. *Radiol. C.I.N. Amer. 18*:117–131, 1980.

22. Knake J. E., Chandler W. F., McGillicuddy J. E., et al. Intraoperative sonography for brain tumor localization and ventricular shunt placement. *A.J.N.R. 3*:425–430, 1982.

23. London D. A., Carroll B. A., and Enzmann D. R. Sonography of ventricular size and germinal matrix hemorrhage in premature infants. *A.J.R. 135*: 559–564, 1980.

24. Mack L. A., Rumack C. M., and Johnson M. L. Ultrasound evaluation of cystic intracranial lesions in the neonate. *Radiology 137*:451–455, 1980.

25. Mack L. A., et al. Intracranial hemorrhage in premature infants: accuracy of sonographic evaluation. *A.J.R. 137*:245–250, 1981.

26. Matsui T., and Hirano A. *An Atlas of The Human Brain for Computerized Tomography.* Tokyo: Igaku-Shoin, 1978.

27. Pape K. E., et al. Ultrasound detection of brain damage in preterm infants. *Lancet 1*:1261–1264, 1979.

28. Rubin J. M., et al. Intraoperative ultrasound examination of the brain. *Radiology 137*:831–832, 1980.
29. Sauerbrei E. E., and Cooperberg P. L. Neonatal brain: sonography of congenital abnormalities. *A.J.N.R. 2*:125–128, 1981.
30. Sauerbrei E. E., et al. Ultrasonic evaluation of neonatal intracranial hemorrhage and its complications. *Radiology 139*:677–685, 1981.
31. Schuman W. P., Rogers J. V., Mack L. A., et al. Real-time sonographic sector scanning of the neonatal cranium. Technique and normal anatomy. *A.J.N.R. 2*:349–356, 1981.
32. Shkolnik A., et al. Intraoperative real-time ultrasonic guidance of ventricular shunt placement in infants. *Radiology 141*:515–517, 1981.
33. *Syllabuses. Perinatal Intracranial Hemorrhage Conference.* Washington, D.C. December 11-13, 1980 and December 2-4, 1982. Publication of Ross Laboratories, Columbus, OH.
34. Volpe J. J. Neonatal intraventricular hemorrhage. *New Engl. J. Med. 304*: 886–891, 1981.

CHAPTER 6

Cross-Sectional and Longitudinal Studies of Brain Stem Auditory-Evoked Potentials in High-Risk Infants

James J. Stockard, M.D., Ph.D.
Janet E. Stockard, B.A.
Allen Merritt, M.D.

This chapter reviews the use of brainstem auditory-evoked potentials (BAEPs) as a diagnostic tool and prognostic indicator in infants at risk for otoneurological impairment in the first year of life. As a diagnostic tool, BAEPs can provide information about the presence, nature, location, and degree of dysfunction in the developing auditory nervous system. When performed serially (longitudinally), the test can answer prognostic questions such as whether the diagnosed otoneurological dysfunction is chronic vs. transient or static vs. evolving and, if evolving, whether it is progressive or resolving. Serial BAEP studies also allow monitoring of the efficacy of any therapeutic interventions.

The key to extracting the maximal amount of clinically useful information from this test begins with the recognition that there are four main types of BAEP abnormalities which have well defined clinical and anatomic correlates and that these abnormalities can each be looked at in two ways—cross-sectionally and longitudinally. These four types of abnormalities will be designated as: (1) Type A central, (2) Type B central, (3) Type I peripheral, and (4) Type II peripheral abnormalities. These four types of abnormalities were initially described—and their clinical correlates defined—in another

---

Perinatal Neurology and Neurosurgery. Edited by R. A. Thompson, J. R. Green, and S. D. Johnsen. Copyright © 1985 by Spectrum Publications, Inc.

article by us [1], which should be referred to for those clinical and methodologic details which are not included in this chapter.

Also, for purposes of clarity, each of the four types of BAEP abnormalities will be discussed first in its routine, cross-sectional application. Only one of these types of abnormalities, the Type A central, will be looked at with the longitudinal perspective afforded by serial studies. The clinical correlates of these four types of abnormalities will be shown in a cross-sectional study of 65 infants at high risk for otological (audiological) and neurological sequelae of a variety of perinatal insults. The infants represent a subgroup from a larger published study [1], which should be consulted for the technical and clinical details. All 65 of the infants in the report had some type of BAEP abnormality.

TYPE A CENTRAL ABNORMALITY— INTERPEAK LATENCY PROLONGATION

BAEP components (waves) I and V are generated in the auditory nerve and rostral brainstem, respectively [2-4], and the interval between these waves (the I–V interpeak latency or I–V IPL) is widely regarded as an indirect measure of "central transmission time" between cochlear nerve and rostral brainstem levels of the auditory pathway. This is an oversimplification, but suffice it to say that the I–V IPL does largely reflect central auditory conduction from neural through brainstem segments of the pathway when there is an intact and normally functioning cochlea. Functional integrity of the basal portions of the cochlea subserving high frequency hearing is especially important to the interpretation of I–V IPL as a "central," or retrocochlear, BAEP measure.

The measurement of a normal I-V IPL is shown in Figure 1, and abnormally prolonged I–V IPLs in cases of Chiari malformation and perinatal asphyxia, respectively, are shown in Figures 2 and 3. A large number of "non-pathologic" physiological and technical factors can greatly affect IPLs in the absence of any neurological dysfunction. These factors must be controlled if IPL interpretation is to be clinically meaningful, and they are reviewed in detail elsewhere [5-11]. Although beyond the scope of this discussion, these non-neurological explanations of IPL prolongation must be excluded before an IPL abnormality can be interpreted as reflecting central auditory conduction disturbance [5-11].

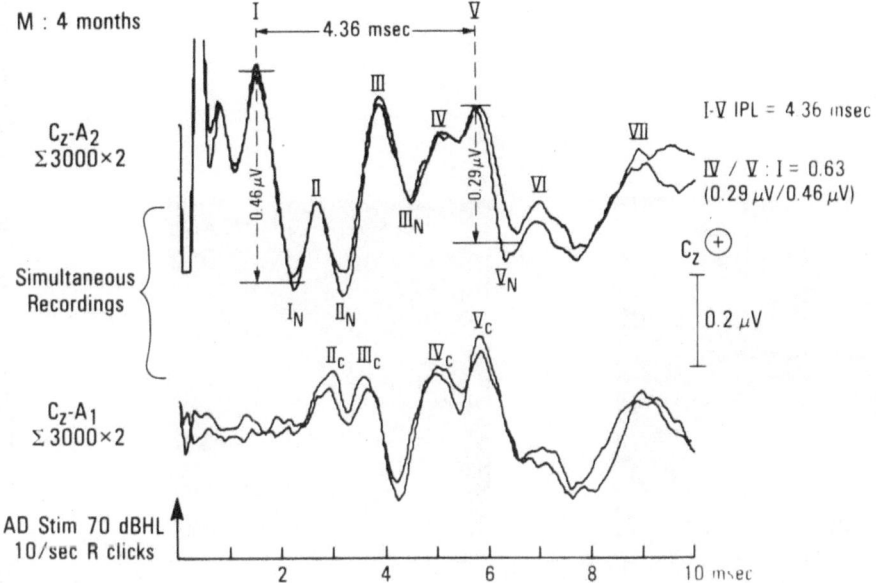

Figure 1. Measurement of I-V IPL and IV/V:I amplitude ratios in a normal infant. Two averages to at least 2048 stimuli were superimposed in this and all subsequent figures to demonstrate response reliability. The IV/V:I amplitude ratio in this case equals 0.63 (0.29 μV/0.46 μV). The pair of tracings recorded simultaneously between the vertex and ear contralateral to acoustic stimulation (Cz-A$_1$ here) is used to allow positive identification of BAEP components [5].

Table 1 includes our criteria for I-V IPL abnormality and Table 2 shows the clinical significance, that is, the otoneurological correlates of that abnormality in long-term follow-up studies. The I-V IPL was considered prolonged when it exceeded our 99% tolerance limit for normal and when wave I was symmetrically normal from both ears or normal from the ear for which the IPL was prolonged. Several preterm infants who were clinically normal on follow-up had *transient* IPL prolongations, but the IPLs had normalized at term in all of these infants. I-V IPL abnormality therefore refers to *persistent* prolongation beyond the age-appropriate 99% tolerance limit for this measure.

As can be seen in Table 2, persistent IPL prolongations were found in the responses from one or both ears in 24 (37%) of the

J. J. Stockard, J. E. Stockard, and A. Merritt

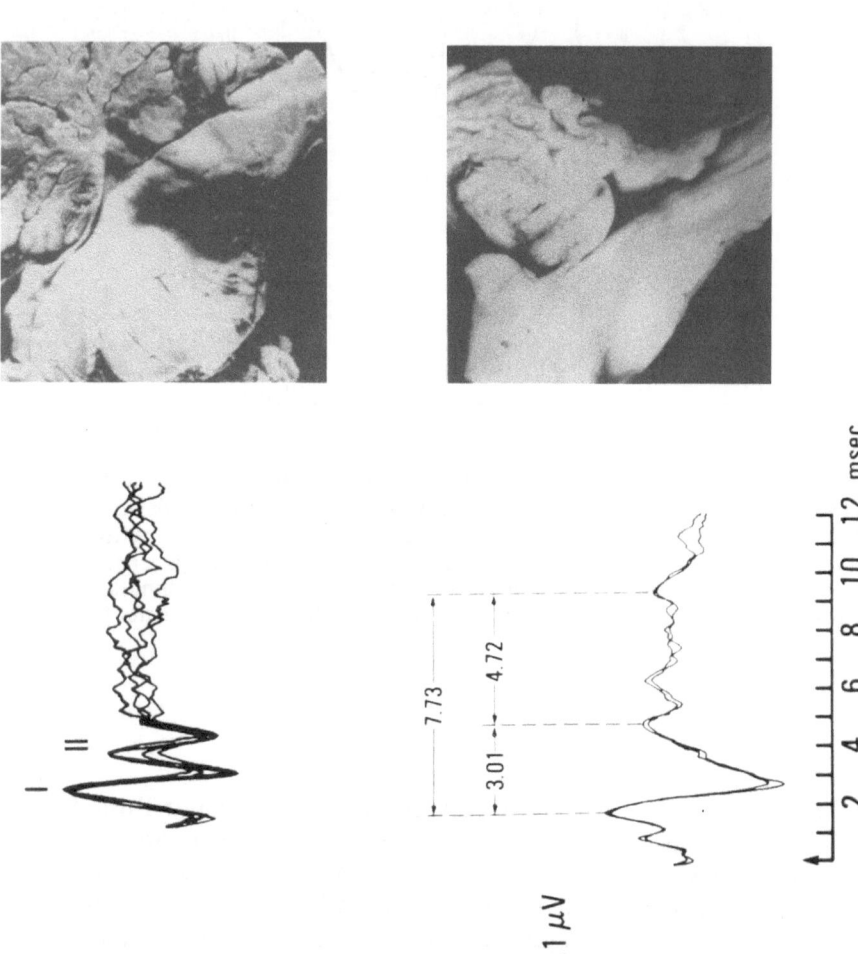

Figure 2.   Two types of central BAEP abnormalities—Type A, with I-V and III-V IPL prolongation due to a Chiari malformation is shown below. Top tracings show absence of later BAEP components (after wave II) in a case of pontine hemorrhage. The IV/V:I AR equals zero in the Type B abnormality shown at top.

Fullterm female: age 2 days
Asphyxia, seizures

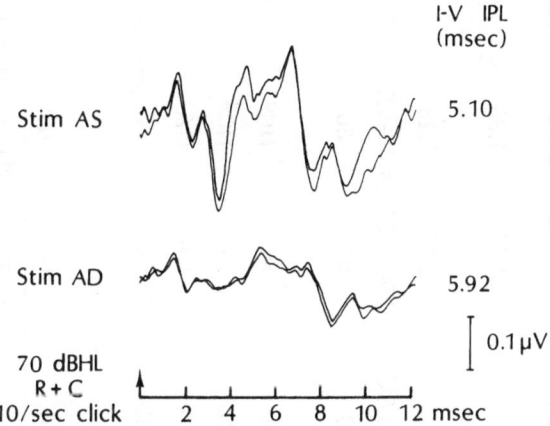

Figure 3. Prolonged I-V and I-III IPLs from the right ear (AD) of an asphyxiated newborn. Abnormal increases in I-V IPL, either bilaterally or unilaterally
and mainly due to prolongations of the I-III response segment, are common in
asphyxia neonatorum. This BAEP abnormality correlates with the selective
vulnerability of the cochlear nuclei and its projections of anoxia/ischemia and
hyperbilirubinemia, as shown in several of our autopsied cases. (Reprinted with
permission from Stockard, J. E., and Stockard J. J. Recording and analyzing. In:
Bases of Auditory Brainstem Evoked Responses, edited by E. Moore. New York:
Grune and Stratton, 1982.)

65 high-risk infants we studied. Of these 24 with Type A central
abnormalities, seven died of causes related to perinatal asphyxia and
13 (76%) of the 17 survivors had gross neurological deficits or
moderate-to-severe psychomotor retardation. Thus, only four (under
one quarter) of the 17 infants with Type A central abnormalities
survived without evidence of major neurological impairment in
clinical follow-up studies. Also, none of the 15 surviving infants who
showed Type A central abnormalities on initial testing had evidence
in audiological follow-up studies of any type of peripheral auditory
dysfunction. Therefore, the Type A central abnormality appears
somewhat sensitive and relatively specific in predicting neurological

Table 1. Normative BAEP Values for Full-term Newborns and Criteria for Classification of BAEP Abnormalities[a]

BAEP Characteristics	Wave I Latency, ms (SI, 110 dBpeSPL)[b]	Wave V L-I Function Slope, μs/dB (SI, 70-110) dBpeSPL	BAEP Threshold dBpeSPL	Wave I Threshold dBpeSPL	Wave V Latency, ms (SI, 110 dBpeSPL)	I-V IPL, ms (SI, 110 dBpeSPL)	IV/V:I AR SI, 110 dBpeSPL	IV/V:I AR SI, 70 dBpeSPL
Normal values								
Mean	1.81	36	≤70 (All subjects)[c]	...	6.72	4.90	0.72	1.13
SD	0.22	7	...	...	0.32	0.28	0.33	0.53
Range	1.48-2.52	24-47	...	≤70 to 80[c]	6.04-7.38	4.35-5.54	0.24-1.7	0.45-2.5
n	55	30	30	30	55	60	30	30
Abnormalities								
Type I, peripheral	Prolonged	WNL	Elevated	NC	NC	NC[d]	WNL	WNL
Type II, peripheral	NC	NC[e]	Elevated	≥110[f]	NC	NC[d]	NC	NC
No response	NA	NA	No response[g]	NA	NA	NA	NA	NA
IPL prolongation	WNL	WNL	WNL	WNL	Prolonged	Prolonged	NC	NC
Absence of later components or AR abnormality	NC	NA	≤90	≤90	NA	NA	<Normal	<Normal

[a] BAEP indicates brainstem auditory evoked potential; SI, stimulus intensity; dBpeSPL, peak equivalent sound pressure level in decibels; L-I, latency-intensity; I-V IPL, interpeak latency (IPL) between waves I and V; IV/V:I AR, amplitude ratio (AR) of wave IV/V to wave I; WNL, within normal limits; NC, no criterion (may be either normal or abnormal); and NA, not applicable.

[b] Because of the prevalence of otitis media and secondary conductive hearing impairment in otherwise normal newborns, subjects with interaural wave I latency asymmetry (difference >0.3 ms) were excluded from the normative data analysis.

[c] Lowest SI delivered to most subjects was 70 dBpeSPL.

[d] These values may be below the normal range.

[e] These values may be above or below normal or WNL.

[f] Response was usually absent at all intensities.

[g] SI was as high as 125 dBpeSPL.

Table 2. Clinical Outcome in Patients With BAEP Abnormalities in the Neonatal Period[a]

Outcome	Absence of Later Components of Abnormal AR	IPL Prolongation	IPL Prolongation With Type II, Peripheral	No Response	Type II, Peripheral	Type I, Peripheral
Normal	...	4 A	...	...	...	2 A-H
Neurologic-developmental abnormalities						
Minimal	...	...	...	...	...	1 A
Moderate-severe	5 (1 A-H, 4 CA)	11 (3 A, 2 H, 6 CA)	...	3 (1 A, 1 H, 1 A-H)	...	3 (1 A-H, 2 CA)
Neurologic abnormalities						
Minimal; SN loss	1 A	...	...	...	...	...
Moderate-severe; SN loss	2 (1 A, 1 CA)	...	2 A	3 (1 A, 1 H, 1 CA)	3 (1 A-H, 1 H, 1 CA)	...
Death	6 (2 A, 2 CA, 1 A-H, 1 IE)	2 A	5 (1 A, 4 CA)	3 (2 A, 1 CA)	2 (1 A-H, 1 CA)	7 (3 A, 4 CA)
SN loss only	...	...	...	...	1 A-H	...
Conductive loss[b]	...	...	...	...	...	8(5A, 1 CA, 2 A-H)

[a]BAEP indicates brainstem auditory potential; AR, amplitude ratio; IPL, interpeak latency; A, asphyxia; A-H, asphyxia-hyperbilirubinemia; CA, congenital anomalies; H, intracranial hemorrhage; SN, sensorineural; and IE, inborn error.
[b]The conductive loss category included patients with and without neurologic abnormalities.

morbidity and mortality, the former seen in three quarters (13/17) of infants with this abnormality who survived long enough for adequate follow-up (two to four years).

TYPE B CENTRAL ABNORMALITY—REDUCED AMPLITUDE OR ABSENCE OF LATER RESPONSE COMPONENTS

Comparison of the amplitude of wave IV/V to that of wave I, as in Figure 1, or of the IV/V amplitude to that of the complex formed by fusion of waves I and II, as shown in Figure 4, provides similar information about central auditory conduction to IPL measurements. When both later and early BAEP components have measurable amplitudes, the amplitude ratio (AR) of the former to the latter is quantified as the IV/V:I (or IV/V:I/II) AR. An example of an abnormal AR is shown in Figure 4, and Table 1 and Figure 5 provide more information about how this selective AR abnormality, or Type B central pattern, is defined. Proper use of AR norms

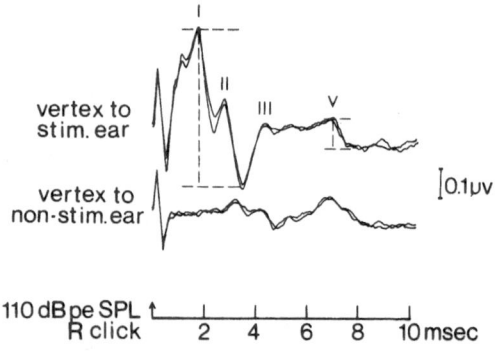

Figure 4. Illustration of IV/V:I/II AR measurement in a premature infant at 45-week conceptional age who had had perinatal hypoxia, hyperbilirubinemia, sepsis and a CT scan consistent with leukoencephalopathy. The vertex-to-nonstimulated-ear recording confirms [5] the identity of the second wave in the routine (vertex-to-stimulated-ear) derivation as a true wave II—rather than bifid wave I. The IV/V:I/II AR measures out to less than 0.2 in this case and this small ratio persisted despite use of higher stimulus rates and lower stimulus intensities. (Reprinted with permission from Stockard, J. E., Stockard, J. J., and Coen, R. W. Auditory brainstem response variability in infants. *Ear and Hearing* 4:11-23, 1983.)

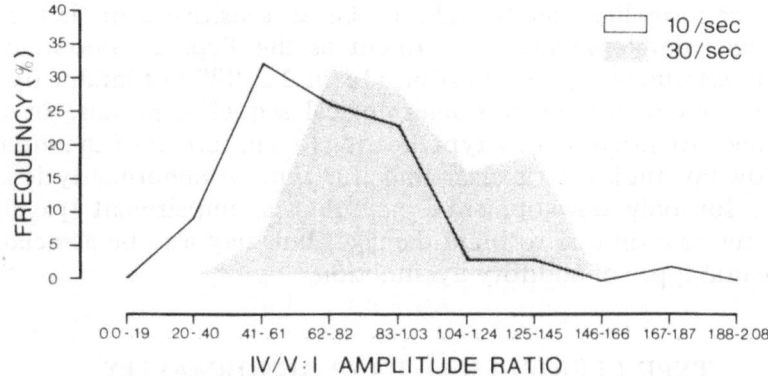

Figure 5. Distributions of IV/V:I/II ARs in term newborns in responses to 10-second and 30-second stimulation with 110 dBpeSPL rarefaction clicks. (Reprinted with permission from Stockard, J. E., Stockard, J. J., and Coen, R. W. Auditory brainstem response variability in infants. *Ear and Hearing 4*: 11–23, 1983.)

requires control for even more physiological and technical variables than does use of IPLs, and, because of this and the non-Gaussian distribution of normal AR values (Figure 5), an AR value should be considered abnormal only if it falls below the entire range of normal shown in Figure 5—given that exactly the same recording technique is employed and patients and controls are age-matched.

When the later response components are immeasurably small, as in the top tracings of Figure 2, and the early components are present, this is still considered an AR abnormality with a value of zero. Using this inclusive definition of Type B central abnormality to cover both quantifiable, finite AR abnormalities and the complete absence of later BAEP waves (AR = 0), our general criteria for defining this type of abnormality are given in Table 1. This table provides the range of values from our control population using the specified stimulus parameters; as mentioned, AR values less than the lower end of this range and down to and including zero are required to ascertain a Type B central abnormality.

As shown in Table 2, 14 (22%) of the 65 high-risk infants we studied had this type of abnormality and, of these 14, 13 (93%) either died or were severely impaired neurologically in follow-up studies. Seven of the eight survivors had moderate-to-severe neurological impairment and three of the eight had minimal-to-moderate sensorineural hearing loss as sequelae (Table 2). Thus the Type B central abnormality can be said to be as sensitive a predictor of neurologic—developmental impairment as the Type A abnormality, with an extremely high proportion (13 of 14, 93%) of infants dying or having moderate-to-severe neurological sequelae. Because of the occurrence of sensorineural-type hearing loss in several of the infants in follow-up studies, it is clear that this type of abnormality is not specific for only developmental neurological impairment (psycho-motor retardation due to brain damage) but may also be associated with neural types of auditory dysfunction.

TYPE I PERIPHERAL BAEP ABNORMALITY

This pattern includes prolongation of wave I latency for the stimulus intensity employed, minimal-to-moderate elevation of the intensity threshold for eliciting waves I and V (Table 1), and normal or "supranormal" central BAEP measures. The I-V IPLs may be shorter than normal and IV/V:I ARs higher than normal due to the greater susceptibility of wave I than wave V to the latency prolongation and amplitude reduction associated with the effective reduction of stimulus intensity, which causes this type of abnor-mality. The specific clinical correlate of the Type I peripheral abnor-mality is conductive-type peripheral hearing loss (Table2).

In addition to the features of Type I abnormality mentioned above, a very important distinguishing feature of this pattern is its association with a normal latency-intensity (L-I) function slope, which helps differentiate it from the Type II peripheral abnormality discussed later (Table 2). Figure 6 shows this and the other character-istics of the Type I peripheral abnormality in a case of unilateral conductive hearing loss due to atresia of the external auditory meatus on one side. In the response from the affected side, wave I latency is prolonged at all stimulus intensities and the threshold for eliciting BAEPs is elevated 20 dB compared to the normal ear. Note, however, that for the intensities at which BAEPs are elicitable, the latencies of waves I and V increase as a function of decreasing stimulus intensity *at the same rate* (that is, with the same L-I slope) as they do from the good ear. This type of parallel L-I function shift is shown graphically in Figure 7 by the "conductive loss" curve, which is characteristic of L-I functions in Type I peripheral abnormalities— showing prolonged latencies of waves at each intensity but *normal rate of latency increase with decreasing stimulus intensity*.

Fullterm female: age 4 days

Goldenhar's syndrome, atresia left external auditory meatus

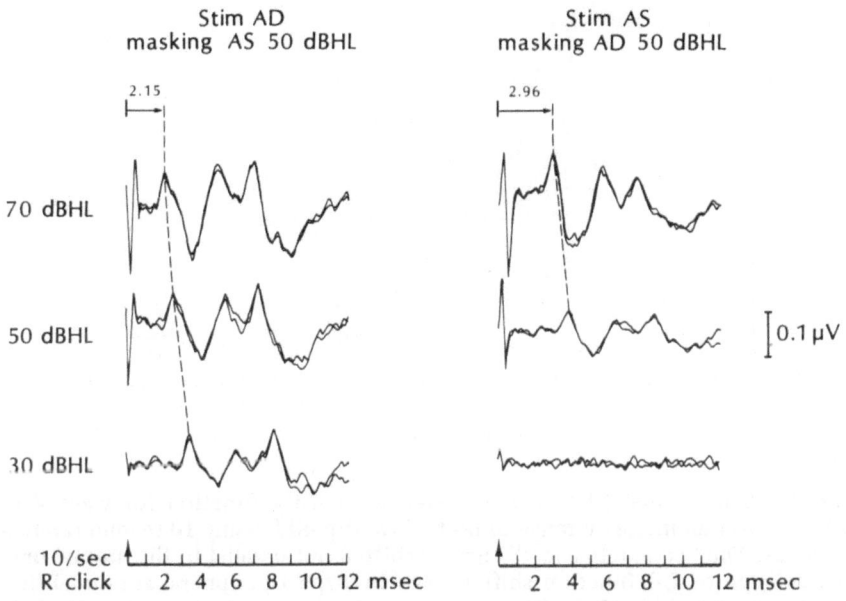

Figure 6. Goldenhar's syndrome, or oculo-auriculo-vertebral dysplasia. A BAEP intensity series is shown which reveals a Type I peripheral abnormality from the left ear (AS). The finding of this abnormality, in turn, indicated the presence of a functional inner ear in this case, which was important information since the inner ear may be either functional or non-functional in this syndrome. BAEP evidence of a functional inner ear allowed simple surgical re-establishment of the patency of the external auditory meatus to restore normal hearing to the ear. (Reprinted with permission from Stockard, J. E., and Stockard, J. J. Recording and analyzing. In: *Bases of Auditory Brainstem Evoked Responses*, edited by E. Moore. New York: Grune and Stratton, 1982.)

This Type I peripheral abnormality is seen commonly as a transient abnormality in small preterm infants, in whom it resolves spontaneously in a large proportion. Persistent Type I peripheral abnormalities were seen in 21 (32%) of our 65 high-risk infants (Table 2) and correlated with conductive hearing loss and serious middle ear disease in more than half of the surviving infants in audiological follow-up studies. Persistent Type I abnormality in the neonatal period puts the infant at especially high risk for chronic serous

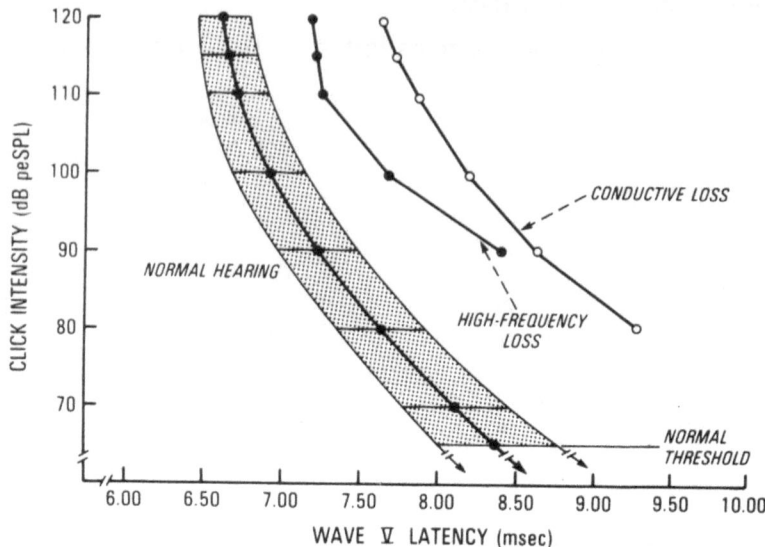

Figure 7. The normal (shaded area) latency-intensity function for wave V in newborns over an intensity range of 65 to 115 dBpeSPL using 10-second rarefaction clicks. The "conductive loss" curve is shifted out parallel to the normal one, and this type of L-I function shift is seen in Type I peripheral abnormalities. The non-parallel shift of the "high-frequency loss" curve is most characteristic of sensorineural deficits and goes along with Type II peripheral abnormalities.

otitis media, and the finding of this pattern on serial BAEP testing should alert pediatricians to this possibility. On the other hand, up to one third of premature infants may show this pattern as only a transient abnormality (Figure 8) when they are retested at term; this pattern of resolving Type I abnormality has no pathological significance. Repeat testing at term or within a month of the initial BAEP study will reveal spontaneous repair of the deficit, as reflected in the BAEP studies of Figure 8.

TYPE II PERIPHERAL BAEP ABNORMALITY

This pattern of BAEP abnormality includes the following: (1) absence or marked threshold elevation of wave I; (2) threshold elevation of wave IV/V; (3) normal or prolonged peak latencies, especially of wave I; (4) normal or abnormally short IPLs, the latter as in Type I abnormality; and (5) latency-intensity functions for

30 week gestation female

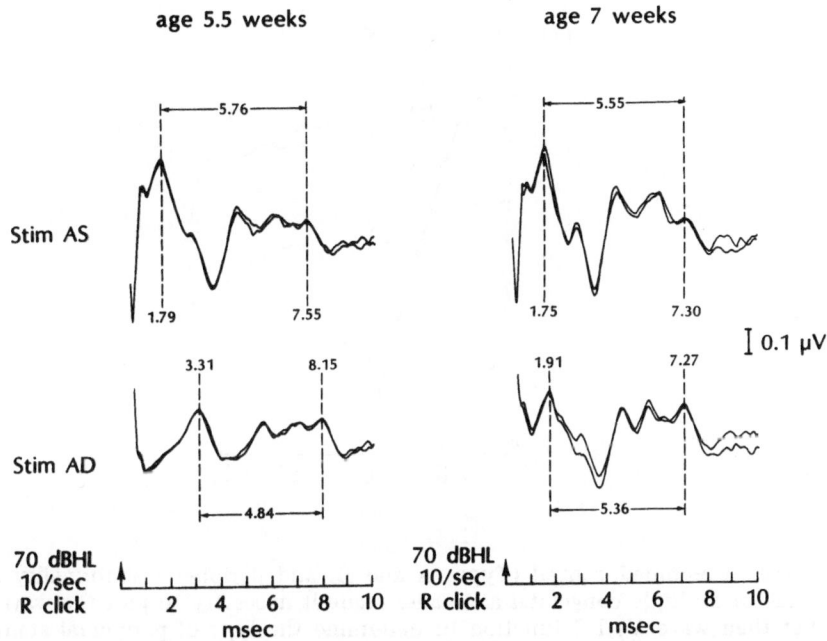

Figure 8. This normal premature infant's BAEPs showed a Type I peripheral abnormality from the right ear (AD) at age 5.5 weeks with a prolongation of wave I latency and an unusually short-for-age I-V IPL from the right ear. Ten days later, after which the infant's weight had increased from 1320 to 1460 gm, wave I latency from the right ear decreased and the I-V IPL *increased* accordingly to a value more consistent with the infant's conceptional age. This infant had been intubated for over a week earlier in her hospital course, and this (intubation) is a common cause of transient Type I abnormality. (Reprinted with permission from Stockard, J. E., and Westmoreland, B. F. Technical considerations in the recording and interpretation of the brainstem auditory evoked potential for neonatal neurologic diagnosis. *Am. J. EEG Technol. 21*:31-54, 1981.)

waves I and/or V which usually diverge from normal (Figures 9 and 10). The last criterion of divergent L-I functions is often useful in distinguishing this pattern of abnormality from the Type I peripheral abnormality since the other criteria for the two types of peripheral abnormality show considerable overlap. The most common direction of L-I function divergence in Type II abnormalities is shown by the

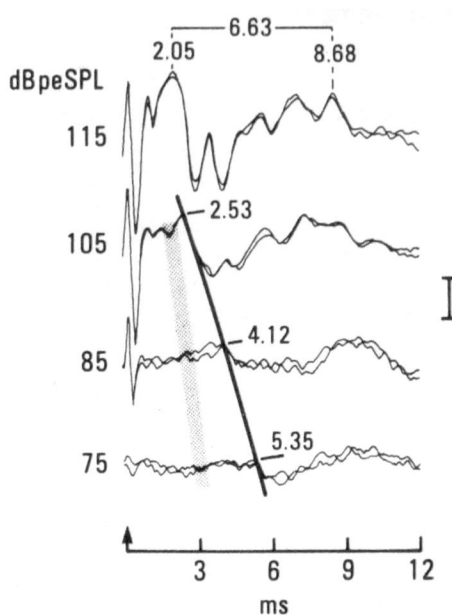

Figure 9. Combined central (Types A and B) and peripheral abnormality in this case of multiple congenital anomalies made it necessary to plot the wave I (rather than wave V) L-I function to determine the type of peripheral abnormality. As can be seen, the rapid divergence of wave I from the normal L-I slope for this wave (shaded area) indicates that this was a Type II, sensorineural-type peripheral abnormality rather than a conductive loss due to any cranial anomalies. Wave V L-I functions are unreliable for the classification of peripheral auditory dysfunction when there are co-existent central BAEP abnormalities. (Reproduced with permission from Stockard, J. E., and Stockard, J. J. Brainstem auditory evoked potentials in normal and otoneurogically impaired newborns and infants. In: *Current Clinical Neurology*, edited by C. Henry. New York: Elsevier Science Publishing Co., 1981.)

curve designated "high-frequency loss" in Figure 7 and exemplified by actual recordings shown in Figures 9 and 10. These intensity series show an increased rate of latency increase for waves I and V as a function of decreasing stimulus intensity; Figure 9 shows the abnormally high L-I slope for wave I and Figure 10 shows it for wave V.

Our normal *mean* L-I slope between 110 and 70 dBpeSPL intensities, using 10-second broad-band rarefaction clicks, is −36 μsec/dB with s.d = 7 μsec/dB and range of −24 to −47 μsec/dB. The occurrence, especially unilaterally, of mean L-I slopes exceeding

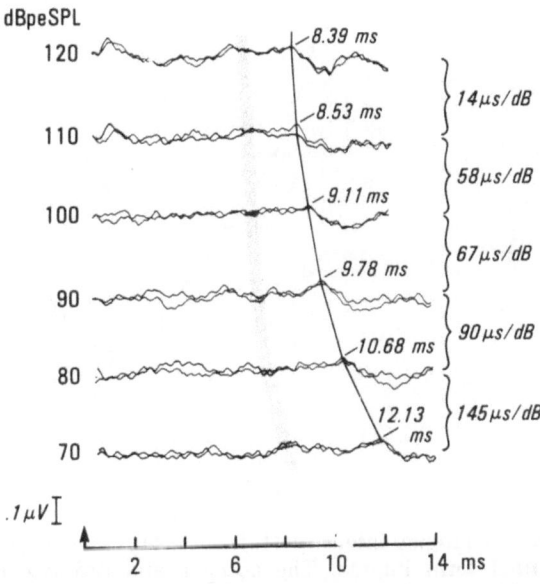

Figure 10. Type II peripheral abnormality showing divergence of wave V L-I curve from normal (shaded area). Note extremely high segmental L-I slopes in low-intensity portions of curve. Neural auditory dysfunction secondary to hypoxic ischemic damage was invoked to explain the Type II abnormality in this case, and later evidence of retrocochlear, sensorineural-type hearing loss was found on audiometric follow-up in this case. (Reprinted with permission from Stockard, J. E., and Stockard, J. J. Brainstem auditory evoked potentials in normal and otoneurologically impaired newborns and infants. In: *Current Clinical Neurophysiology*, edited by C. Henry. New York: Elsevier Science Publishing Co., 1981.)

–55 μsec/dB is regarded as supportive of a Type II pattern of abnormality when the other criteria are present. In this context, it is important to realize the non-linearity of the *normal* L-I function over the 65 to 115 dB peSPL intensity range usually tested, as illustrated in Figure 11. As is clear from Figure 11, the validity of any mean L-I slope between intensities at the extremes of this range could conceivably reflect a few intensity segments which are either markedly abnormal or absent (as in the case of miscalibrated stimulus intensities coming out of the headphone). The "mean" L-I slope can easily be rendered falsely normal or abnormal if one is operating in a different intensity range than one assumes, since there will be disproportional weighting of high L-I slope values in the low-intensity segments and

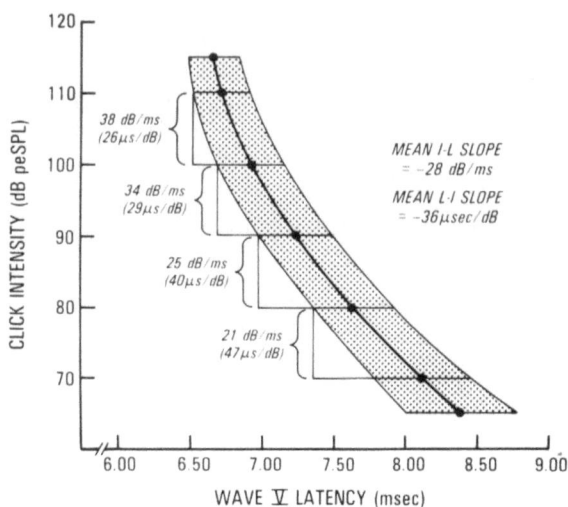

Figure 11. Normal latency-intensity (L-I)/intensity-latency (I-L) function for wave V in normal term infants. The abscissa and ordinate for this plot are reversed from what is seen elsewhere in the literature to facilitate comparison with the actual BAEP intensity series as they are recorded. Note the marked differences in the segmental L-I/(I-L) slopes from each other, and from the mean slopes for the entire curve, depending on what intensity range one is operating in.

disproportionate contributions of low L-I values if the high-intensity segments are overrepresented (Figure 11).

Type II abnormalities occurred in 13 (20%) of our high-risk infants and occurred in combination with IPL prolongation in seven of these (Table 2). As can be seen in Table 2, seven of the 13 infants with this type of abnormality expired and all of the remaining six survivors had sensorineural hearing losses in audiological follow-up studies. This type of abnormality is thus highly correlated with cochlear-retrocochlear hearing loss, usually of the high-frequency and, sometimes, recruiting type. Its association with a high prevalence of clinical or BAEP evidence of co-existent central nervous system injury is not surprising given the shared selective vulnerability of extra-axial and intra-axial auditory nervous system structures to perinatal asphyxia and its concomitants [12-15].

LONGITUDINAL ANALYSIS OF TYPE A CENTRAL ABNORMALITIES IN INFANTS AT RISK

To this point, we have dealt with four types of cross-sectional BAEP abnormalities, that is, abnormality defined by taking latency and amplitude values or latency-intensity and amplitude-intensity (threshold) functions and comparing them with a population of normal control values all recorded at the same age. One can, instead, take any of the BAEP measures discussed above and look at its development in a single infant and compare its overall maturation to the normal ontogeny of that variable in a control population. This is a much more sensitive way of picking up the brainstem or neural dysfunction reflected in BAEPs since the individual infant serves as his/her own control. Clinical application of this approach to BAEP analysis will now be discussed for one response measure, IPL.

Figure 12 shows the normal logarithmic decrease in I-V IPL from 29-week conceptional age to term in an infant with no known neurological or otological abnormalities, either at the time or in follow-up studies. As can be seen in Figure 12, the average I-V IPL change from week to week (0.4-0.5 msec) is an order of magnitude greater than the standard deviation of the measure itself at any given age (0.04-0.05 msec). This plus the fact that estimates of conceptional age are accurate only to the nearest one to two weeks make it obvious that cross-sectional interpretation of any preterm infant's BAEPs is on somewhat shaky ground. A compounding difficulty in the cross-sectional interpretation of BAEPs in prematurity is the fact that BAEP data from preterm infants without apparent pathology have unpredictable and usually non-Gaussian population distributions. As shown in Figure 13 and 14, IPLs from preterm infants appear to be bimodally distributed, partly along gender lines, with the lower-mode peak containing a predominance of female premature infants ($p < 0.10$). With advancing age, the two peaks tend to converge (Figure 14) until, at term, there is a unimodal (but heterogeneous) Gaussian IPL distribution [11].

For all of the reasons cited in the last paragraph, we consider it unwise to interpret any isolated study in an infant under 36 weeks of conceptional age as pathologically abnormal and of unfavorable prognostic significance. The more prudent and valid approach is to reserve judgment until at least one repeat recording is obtained from the infant when he/she is as old as 38 to 42 weeks conceptional age

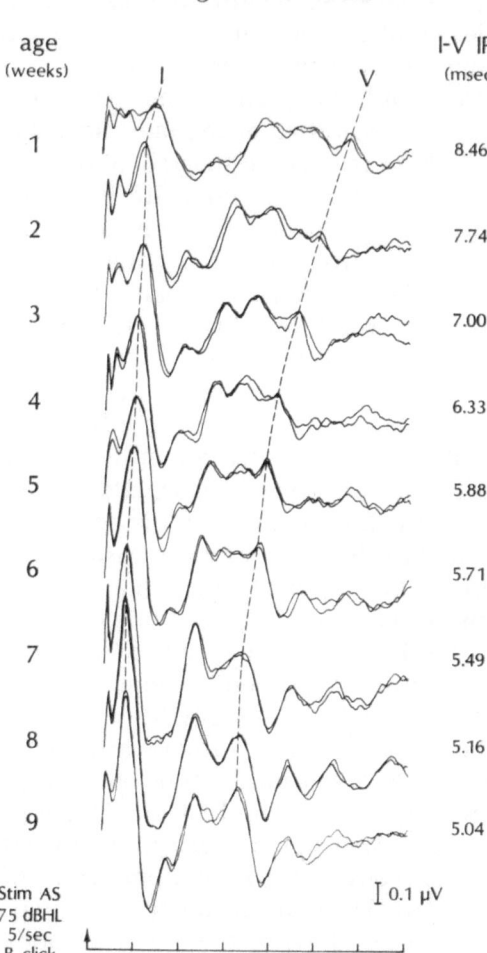

28 week gestation female

Figure 12. Longitudinal BAEP study from a normal infant, from 29 weeks conceptional age through 37 weeks. Note the logarithmic decrease in wave I and wave V latencies, as well as the IPL between these components, and the progressive increase in IV/V:I/II AR with advancing age. (Reproduced with permission from Stockard, J. E., and Westmoreland, B. F. Technical considerations in the recording and interpretation of the brainstem auditory evoked potential for neonatal neurologic diagnosis. *Am. J. EEG Technol.* *21*:31–54, 1981.)

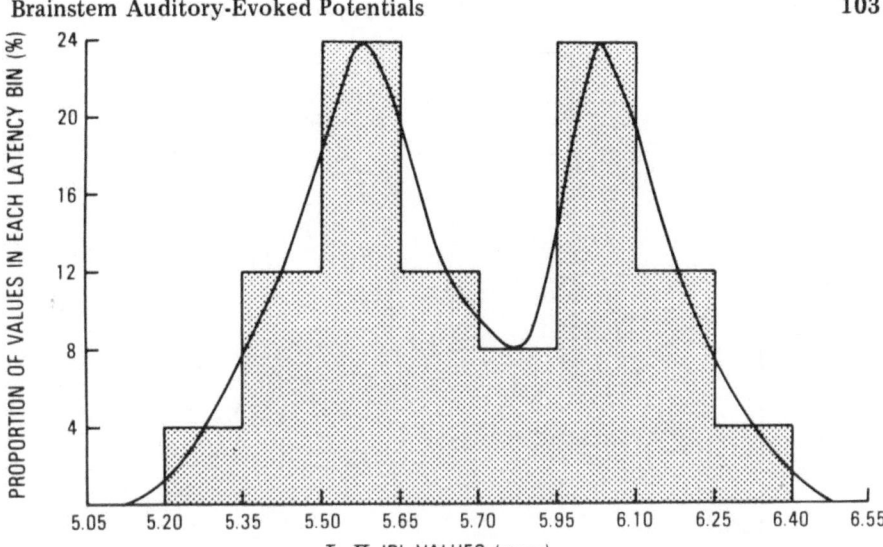

Figure 13. Bimodal distribution of I-V IPLs in our 33- to 34-week conceptional age preterm infants who had no radiologically or clinically manifest abnormality. There was a tendency (p<0.10) for females to group in the lower-mode peak and for males to segregate out into the higher-mode peak. Compare with Figure 14.

(or in lieu of this, a normal follow-up recording at an earlier age). The initial study in early prematurity, if outside of "normal limits," is best considered the first data point for a longitudinal BAEP analysis. Figure 15 illustrates nicely the wisdom of a conservative interpretative approach to even the most extreme examples of apparent BAEP abnormality: at 29 weeks conceptional age, BAEPs were completely absent, but on repeat testing six weeks later they were normal—as was the infant. Thus, unfavorable prognostic significance can be inferred from a BAEP "abnormality" in this age group only if it persists or worsens in longitudinal studies.

The continued logarithmic shortening of IPLs postterm is shown in Figure 16. This figure illustrates the main point of this section—that marked abnormalities of BAEP maturational trends may be revealed by serial studies even though each study, considered in isolation, is within normal limits for the age of the infant when looked at cross-sectionally. The two cases depicted in Figure 16 demonstrate this. The first, designated by the open squares was an infant who began to diverge from the normal age–IPL curve as early as the first month of life, after which he began to have recurrent

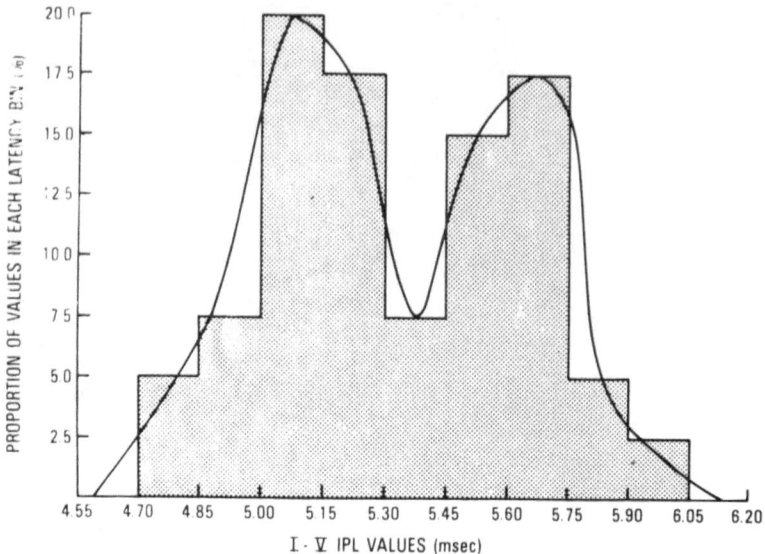

Figure 14. Asymmetrically bimodal I-V IPL distribution in "normal" (that is, without clinically or radiologically manifest pathology) 35- to 37-week conceptional age infants. Note that the two peaks have begun to converge, and that they have lower absolute modal values, compared to the two peaks in the distribution for 33- to 34-week conceptional age infants (Figure 13).

life-threatening apneic episodes requiring resuscitation (Near-Miss-for-Sudden-Infant-Death-Syndrome, or NMSIDS). As seen in Figures 16 and 17, his IPL values stopped diverging from normal at four months of age and were *converging* by six months of age. It was at about this time that the infant stopped having NMSID episodes. Whether the IPL divergence, then convergence, with the normal age–IPL function is more related to the cause or to the effect of the recurrent apneic episodes is another issue under study [16]; nonetheless, the tight electroclinical correlation between IPL divergence and risk-for-apnea which we have observed does have empiric clinical utility.

For example, the other case plotted in Figure 16 (open triangles) was an infant who began to cross age–IPL percentiles between age 9 to 12 months, having had a high-normal but parallel-to-normal age–IPL curve up until that age. It was at the time that his age–IPL trajectory diverged from normal (Figure 16) that the infant began to have progressively severe sleep apneic episodes. At the age of 15 months, after his age–IPL function had clearly diverged sharply from normal, he began to have NMSIDS episodes. Hospitalization for sleep

Premature male: 27 weeks gestation
RDS, hyperbilirubinemia
Normal exam 6 months later

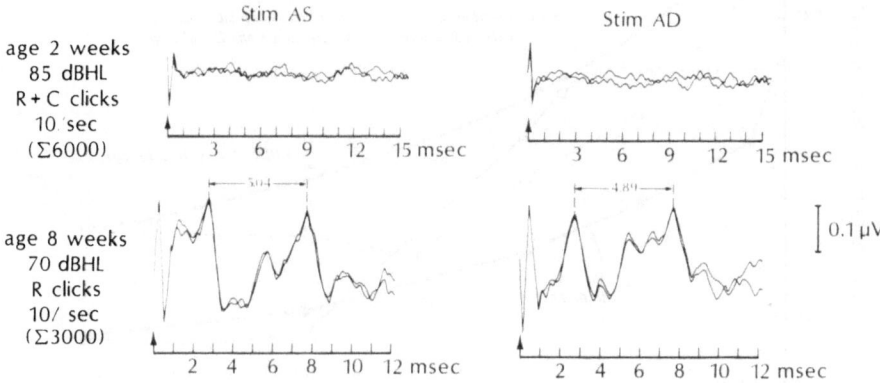

Figure 15. Premature male whose neonatal course was complicated by respiratory distress syndrome and hyperbilirubinemia. Initial BAEP testing showed complete absence of responses bilaterally despite optimal technique. Repeat testing six weeks later showed normal BAEPs and the infant was neurologically and audiologically normal in follow-up studies one year later. See text for further discussion. (Reproduced with permission from Stockard, J. E., and Stockard, J. J. Recording and analyzing. In: *Bases of Auditory Brainstem Evoked Responses*, edited by E. Moore. New York: Grune and Stratton, 1982.)

monitoring and pulmonary studies at that time yielded a negative work-up with no significant apneic events observed. At this point, the longitudinal BAEP divergence from normal age–IPL curves was the only objective evidence of any brainstem dysfunction; the BAEP measures from all studies up to and including that performed at 15 months would have been interpreted as normal if analyzed only in temporal cross-section (Figure 16). Further divergence of the IPL curve to near the age-appropriate upper limit of normal at age 18 months prompted a more intensive evaluation of the infant's continuing tendency to severe, recurrent sleep apnea. This last evaluation revealed evidence of occult Leigh's disease as the etiology of the episodes and provided a basis for treatment.

BAEPs from another similar case, in which arrest of BAEP maturation was the first objective evidence of brainstem dysfunction in an infant with a history of NMSIDS episodes, are shown in Figure 18. Preliminary laboratory studies now indicate that the

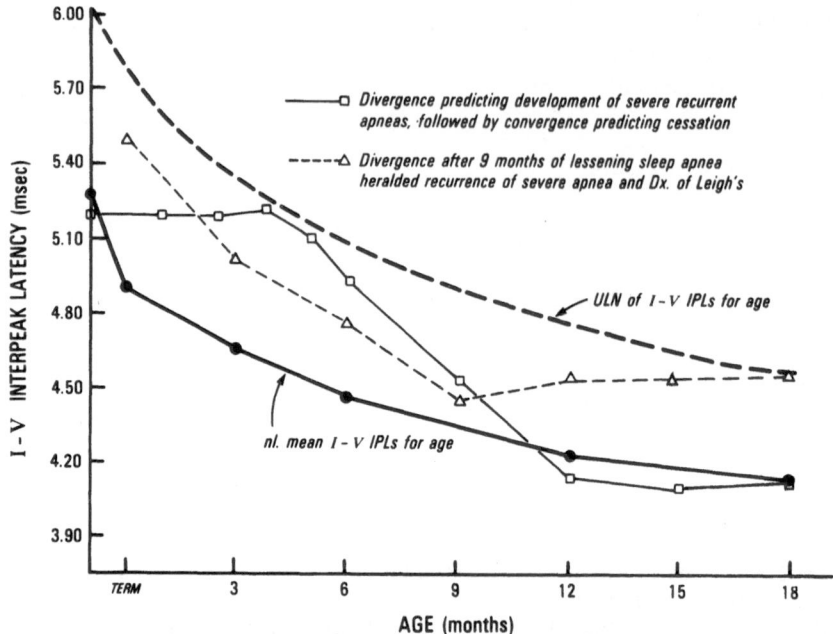

Figure 16. Normal age-IPL function over first 18 months of life, showing both normal mean curve and upper limit of normal curve for values obtained at any given age. The two cases shown by the faint lines connecting open symbols are described in the text.

life-threatening sleep apneic episodes in this case are probably also due to Leigh's disease; high-dose thiamine treatment has been associated with some evidence of *both* clinical and BAEP improvement over the 10 months since administration of vitamin B_1. It should be emphasized that once an identifiable pathogenetic mechanism can be invoked and documented in an infantile apnea syndrome, the syndrome no longer falls into the category of SIDS or NMSIDS, which is—by definition—cryptogenic. Nonetheless, the use of longitudinal BAEP abnormalities to index specific, subsequently identifiable biochemical bases of cases that initially present as "idiopathic" NMSIDS is exciting. The possible role of longitudinal BAEP analysis in identifying infants at risk for SIDS is of special interest now that, after initial enthusiasm [17,18] for the technique, cross-sectional BAEP findings have now convincingly been demonstrated *not* to be markers for risk-of-SIDS [16,19,20]. The hypothesis that longitudinal BAEP abnormalities might be such a marker in some cases needs to be tested.

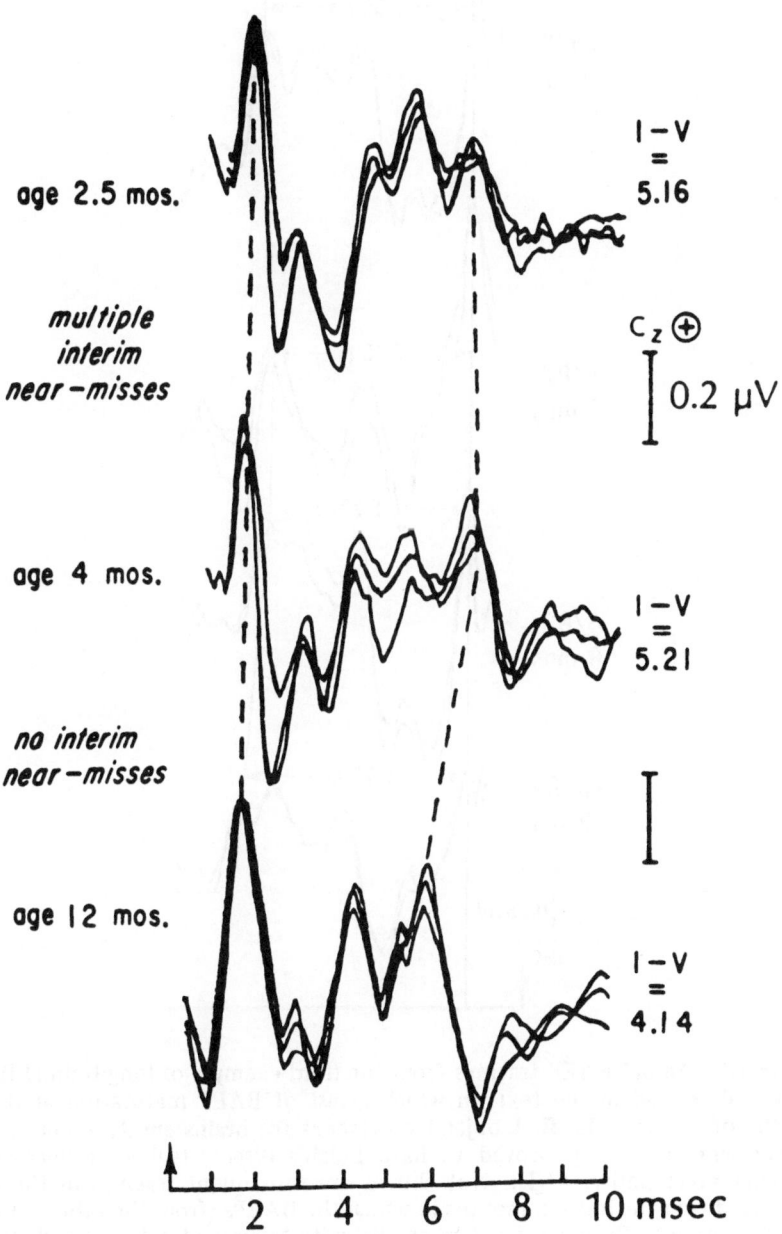

Figure 17. BAEPs from first case described in text and represented by the curve comprised of open squares in Figure 16.

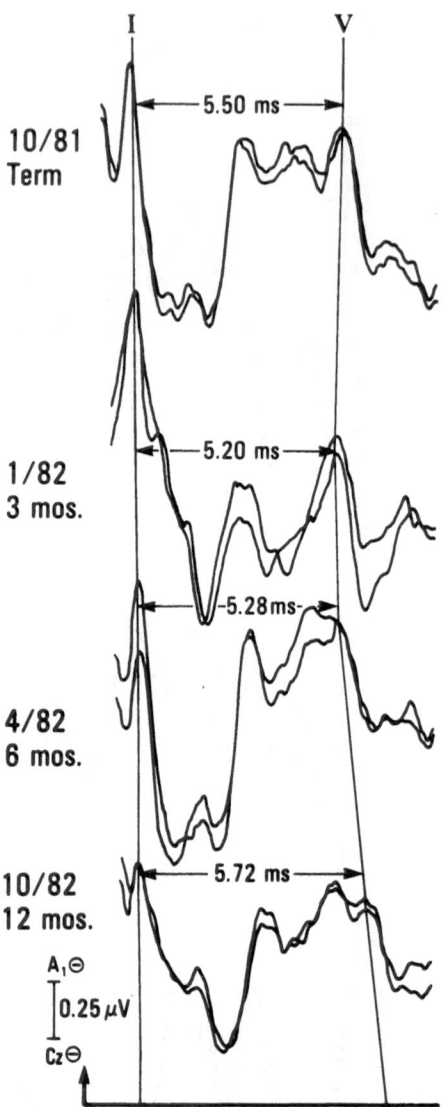

Figure 18. Actual BAEP tracings from the third example of longitudinal BAEP analysis described in the text, in which arrest of BAEP maturation at 3 to 6 months of age was the first objective evidence for brainstem dysfunction in a patient who ultimately proved to have Leigh's disease (subacute necrotizing encephalomyelopathy, SNE). Not shown are subsequent tracings in this case performed over the last ten months in which the BAEPs (from the other ear than that shown) actually *normalized* in parallel with thiamine treatment and clinical improvement. The I-V IPL from the ear studied in the figure has also shown improvement with treatment over this period, decreasing over 1 msec to approximately 4.6 to 4.7 msec.

In summary, we have described four types of BAEP abnormalities in infancy which are sensitive to, and relatively specific for, certain otoneurological conditions that most neonatal intensive care graduates—and virtually all small premature infants—are at risk for. The patterns of abnormality and their clinical correlates are: (1) Type A central—predictive of retrocochlear neural or brain stem dysfunction; (2) Type B central—predictive of sensorineural auditory and brainstem dysfunction; (3) Type I peripheral—predictive of conductive-type peripheral auditory dysfunction; and (4) Type II peripheral—predictive of cochlear or sensorineural-type auditory dysfunction. The latency and amplitude measures or parametric studies (studies of BAEP changes resulting from changing stimulus parameters), used to define these abnormalities in individuals vis-à-vis age-matched control populations in the routine cross-sectional way, can also be looked at longitudinally in serial BAEP studies of the same infant. This latter, newer approach to infant BAEP analysis promises to increase the sensitivity and specificity of the test for pathology of the developing brainstem and hearing apparatus and to allow earlier therapeutic interventions to protect the functions of these critical structures.

ACKNOWLEDGMENTS

The authors are indebted to the Grass Instrument Company for providing the equipment necessary to carry out these studies and to the National Sudden Infant Death Syndrome Foundation, whose funding made this research possible.

REFERENCES

1. Stockard, J. E., Stockard, J. J., Kleinberg, F., and Westmoreland, B. F. Prognostic value of brainstem auditory evoked potentials in neonates. *Arch. Neurol.* 40:360–365, 1983.
2. Stockard, J. J., and Rossiter, V. Clinical and pathologic correlates of brainstem auditory response abnormalities. *Neurology* 27:316–325, 1977.
3. Starr, A., and Hamilton, A. Correlation between confirmed sites of neurological lesions and far-field auditory brainstem responses. *Electroenceph. Clin. Neurophysiol.* 41:595–608, 1976.
4. Stockard, J. J., and Iragui, V. J. Clinically useful applications of evoked potentials in adult neurology. *Journal of Clinical Neurophysiology* 1(2): 159-202, 1984.

5. Stockard, J. J., Stockard, J. E., and Sharbrough, F. W. Nonpathologic factors influencing brainstem auditory evoked potentials. *Am. J. EEG Technol.* *18*:177-200, 1978.
6. Stockard, J. E., Stockard, J. J., Westmoreland, B. F., and Corfits, J. L. Brainstem auditory evoked responses: Normal variation as a function of stimulus and subject characteristics. *Arch. Neurol. 36*:823-831, 1979.
7. Stockard, J. J., Stockard, J. E., and Sharbrough, F. W. Brainstem auditory evoked potentials in neurology: Methodology, interpretation, clinical application. In: *Electrodiagnosis in Clinical Neurology*, edited by M. Aminoff, pp. 370-413. New York: Churchill Livingstone, 1980.
8. Stockard, J. E., and Stockard, J. J. Brainstem auditory evoked potentials in normal and otoneurologically impaired newborns and infants. In: *Current Clinical Neurophysiology*, edited by C. Henry, pp. 421-466. New York: Elsevier Science Publishing Co., 1981.
9. Stockard, J. E., and Westmoreland, B. F. Technical considerations in the recording and interpretation of the brainstem auditory evoked potential for neonatal neurologic diagnosis. *Am. J. EEG Technol. 21*:31-54, 1981.
10. Stockard, J. E., and Stockard, J. J. Recording and analyzing. In: *Bases of Auditory Brainstem Evoked Responses*, edited by E. Moore, pp. 255-286. New York: Grune and Stratton, 1982.
11. Stockard, J. E., Stockard, J. J., and Coen, R. W. Auditory brainstem response variability in infants. *Ear and Hearing 4*:11-23, 1983.
12. Hall, J. On the neuropathological changes in the CNS following perinatal asphyxia. *Acta. Otolaryngol. Suppl. 188*:331-339, 1964.
13. Griffiths, A., and Laurence, K. The effect of hypoxia and hypoglycemia on the brain of the newborn human infant. *Dev. Med. Child Neurol. 16*:308-319, 1974.
14. Gerrard, J. Nuclear jaundice and deafness. *J. Laryngol. Otol. 66*:39-46, 1952.
15. Leech, R. W., and Alvord, E. C. Anoxic-ischemic encephalopathy in the human neonatal period: the significance of brainstem involvement. *Arch. Neurol. 34*:109-113, 1977.
16. Stockard, J. J. Brainstem auditory evoked potentials in adult and infant apnea syndromes, including sudden infant death syndrome (SIDS) and near miss for sudden infant death. *Ann. NY Acad. Sci. 388*:433-465, 1982.
17. Orlowski, J., Nodar, R., and Lonsdale, D. Abnormal brainstem auditory evoked potentials in infants with threatened sudden infant death syndrome. *Cleve. Clin. Q. 46*:77-81, 1979.
18. Nodar, R., Lonsdale, D., and Orlowski, J. Abnormal brainstem potentials in infants with threatened sudden infant death syndrome. *Otolaryngol. Head. Neck. Surg. 88*:619-621, 1980.
19. Gupta, P. R., Guilleminault, C., and Dorfman, L. J. Brainstem auditory evoked potentials in near-miss sudden infant death syndrome. *J. Pediatr. 98*:791-794, 1981.
20. Lueders, H., Orlowski, J., Dinner, D. S., Lesser, R. P. and Klem, G. Far-field auditory evoked potentials in near-miss sudden infant death syndrome. *Arch. Neurol. 41*:615-617, 1984.

CHAPTER 7

Neurosurgery in Congenital Defects Other Than Hydrocephalus

Hector E. James, M.D.

INTRODUCTION

The defects, in general, are quite common and 5 of 100 children are born with a significant abnormality. Considering the complex event that leads to the development of a fetus and subsequently a child, 5% is certainly a low figure.

We will consider, in this topic, disorders of the spine. The spine is primarily involved in the disease because of the location of closure of the fetus into a tube, a complex phenomenon that occurs in the third to fourth week of gestation. The most common disease of this type is spina bifida cystica or myelomeningocele (myelo for spinal cord and meninges for the covering of the cord). It is not a new disease as it has been described as far back as 2000 B.C. Over 6,000 children in the United States are born with this disorder. It occurs in approximately 1 per 1,000 deliveries and, in certain cases or in certain regions, as high as 3 per 1,000 deliveries. This most obvious failure of adequate closure and obvious defect at birth is paralleled by a more occult phenomenon, just as devastating as myelomeningocele if undetected. This other-end-of-the-spectrum disorder has various names: spinal dysrhaphia, the syndrome of spina bifida occulta and/or tethered cord syndrome. See Table 1 for a discussion of terminology.

We will address these groups together initially from the point of view of early detection, early management, and the role of the neonatologist, neonatal nursing, and intensive care unit facility.

Perinatal Neurology and Neurosurgery. Edited by R. A. Thompson, J. R. Green, and S. D. Johnsen. Copyright © 1985 by Spectrum Publications, Inc.

Table 1.   Terminology

1. **Myelomeningocele or spina bifida cystica:**   A disorder of the midline charac-terized by a developmental anomaly of ectoderm, mesoderm, and neuroecto-derm, without cutaneous covering, more commonly located in the lumbosacral region, and causing varying degrees of denervation.

2. **Meningocele:**   A disorder of the midline which characteristically involves the mesoderm and only rarely the neuroectoderm, with intact ectoderm. Thus, the child presents more commonly at the lumbosacral level with a skin-covered mass. There is a bifid defect that can be easily detected radiologically that usually in-volves various segments and presents with absence of lamina and spinous processes.

3. **Spinal dysrhaphia or the syndrome of spina bifida occulta:**   This is a dis-order of the midline that is characterized by varying degrees of involvement of the neuroectoderm and mesoderm with, at times, a cutaneous marker in a skin-covered region. It is more common in the lumbosacral area and is characterized by an insidious and progressive neurological picture involving the lower extrem-ities, bowel and bladder control, or both.

4. **Spinal hamartomas:**   Disorders of the midline in which there are ectopically located mature elements representing various layers of formation. Thus they can be gland, ectopic fat, renal structures, cartilage, and bone located within and out of the spinal canal. There is no neoplastic quality to these, and their importance is that they represent an element in the spectrum of disorders of the midline that can cause neurological problems with time, if they have not already, due to their location.

5. **Teratomas:**   Teratomas represent potentially neoplastic midline changes that are commonly present as a large mass, most often in the sacrococcygeal region. They may involve neural elements, but the more distal they are in the canal, the less likely. They commonly involve the pelvic floor. The neoplastic potential, though initially not evident in the microscopy of the specimen removed in the neonatal period, becomes evident with time if untreated.

DEVELOPMENTAL AND GENETIC ASPECTS

The formation of the fetus is an extremely complex series of events that, from the standpoint of neurological disorders of the mid-line, relate to specific periods in development surrounding the third to fourth week of gestation. At that point, the three basic germinal layers of ectoderm, mesoderm, and entoderm are linked in such a way that the midportion of the ectoderm differentiates into a spe-cific structure by forming a groove on the surface that subsequently will become a tube, as lateral coverage of this tube occurs. This process leads to complete closure of a tube by the fourth week of pregnancy, initiating in the midportion of the fetus and extending simultaneously to the head and to the sacral region. The failure of this closure to occur leads to the process of myelomeningocele or meningocele. The closure that is disordered or that traps the rest of mesoderm or ectoderm within it as it closes will lead to the occult spinal disorders (spinal dysrhaphia).

The reason that developmental problems occur in certain instances is not known. There are multiple theories yet none of them have been proven. There are experimental models to create myelo-dysplasia in animals, such as exposing the animal to external heat on a certain date of the pregnancy. The newborn animals are then often born with defects. Much research is ongoing and certainly more information will be available in time.

There is a familial predisposition to this disorder, though the majority of cases are spontaneous mutations. If a mother bears a child with myelomeningocele, the geneticists inform us that she has a 5% chance of giving birth to another child with a similar problem. Likewise, in families with myelomeningocele, there is a higher incidence of spinal dysrhaphia and vice versa, as documented by recent work.

PHYSIOPATHOLOGY

In the open disorders, such as myelomeningocele, there is a failure of the neural tube to close at the level of the disease, and this creates a lack of adequate migration of the neural elements and consequently poor distal innervation will occur from that particular level. This poor migration and continuous exposure of the neural derivatives during the remainder of the pregnancy will lead to permanent neurological damage of those particular dermatomes affected. The dorsal structures that normally cover the spinal cord have not come into position, the somite has not formed correctly laterally and dorsally, and consequently, the paraspinal muscles and lamina are not in location. This combination of the poorly formed muscle and bone layers as well as the denervation can, in many cases, result in pathological curvatures, sych as a gibbus deformity and scoliosis.

What we have just described is a myelomeningocele or spina bifida cystica. There can be an extremely tenuous rudiment of a membrane trying to cover the defect or there can be no coverage whatsoever. A milder form of disease is manifested by a meningocele. In these situations, the somite and related mesodermal structures do not form normally, but very commonly the neural derivatives are next-to-normal or normal in their location. Thus, the dura, which is involved in the disease process as part of a mesodermal derivative, can be out-pouching through a defect in the lamina and muscle, as a fluid-filled cavity, which is characteristically covered by intact skin. This mass then palpates as a soft mass, and there is a defect of the spinous processes and lamina underneath it. Upon arrival to the neonatal intensive care unit, these children are examined and the results are normal.

The occult disorders may present without any cutaneous visible marking, such as that which seems to occur in about 50% of the cases, and in other cases, there are local changes in the midline, more commonly over the lumbosacral spine, that herald underlying disorders in the formation of these structures. Cutaneous markers, such as a local tuft of hair, deep dimples or local masses in the subcutaneous tissue bulging under the skin, are characteristic of spinal lipomas with a subcutaneous and an intraspinal component. The importance of these findings is that they alert the physician to underlying pathology that needs to be evaluated further. This pathology may be arachnoidal bands and scarring on nerve roots and the spinal cord, dermoid or epidermoid cysts, or spinal lipomas as previously related. These may then cause neurological damage during gestation or continue to do do in the postnatal life.

Normally during development, there is a disproportionate growth between the bony spinal canal and the neural elements in the spinal cord. Thus, the spinal bony canal grows at a far more rapid rate than the spinal cord, and, since the spinal cord is attached to the cervical-medullary junction, the spinal cord has a relative upward migration within the bony canal as this increases in length. This upward migration is permitted by an involution of the distal portion of the spinal cord into a thin, two mm gliotic structure, which is attached to the lower portion of the dorsal sacral bodies, the filum terminale. In certain conditions, the filum does not involute, remains thick and anchors the distal portion of the functional cord, the conus, and creates a distraction as it is normally meant to be migrating upwards. Called the tethering effect, this distraction creates the progressive denervation of the lower spinal nerve roots. In other situations, the dermoid cysts, lipomas, or arachnoidal bands and scar formation anchor themselves to the nerve roots or conus thus creating the limitation of upward migration, and causing the tethering effect. Finally, masses such as lipomas or dermoid cysts growing inside a rigid or semirigid bony enclosure can cause progressive pressure on the spinal cord or neural elements and thus create the dysfunction. This is known as the compressive form of physiopathology.

Other disorders that subsequently enter into the differential diagnosis which are important to keep in mind in evaluating a child with a spinal mass, are the midline teratomas more commonly located in the sacrococcygeal region. Often they are grotesque masses that are easily diagnosed by their enormous appearance at birth. These, at that point in time, usually are made of mature elements located out of place and do not have specific neoplastic potential if totally removed at that time. On the other hand, these can degenerate if untreated. Another group of disorders of the midline that can present as less visible masses, which are located anywhere along the midline, are the spinal hamartomas. They are truly masses of mature elements of the various layers that originally formed the fetus with no neoplastic characteristics, and they do not enter the category of true teratomas by their cytology. They should, however, be treated as any other spinal dysrhaphia since they may create neurological damage because of their location.

In myelomeningoceles and in spinal dysrhaphia, the most common location for the disorder is in the lumbosacral region. Thoracolumbar disorders then follow in frequency and the least common are the cervical ones. The complete opening of the spine because of total failure of closure is extremely rare and incompatible with more than a few hours of life. This is termed rachischisis. If this disorder involves the cranium, it is called anencephaly. Likewise, this is incompatible with life. These extremes are not as common as the lumbosacral myelomeningoceles and dysrhaphic conditions. Proportionally, meningoceles are less common than myelomeningoceles.

There are other disorders of the formation of the central nervous system in myelomeningoceles. Thus, possibly due to migration of the neural elements, a maldevelopment can occur along the midline of the intracranial portion of the central nervous system that can lead either to a maldevelopment of the aqueduct of Sylvius, such as forking (two or more channels instead of one aqueduct, the overall surface is not sufficient to pass the required cerebrospinal fluid through it) or a caudal and dorsal migration of the hindbrain and cerebellum, creating an impaction of the same in the low posterior fossa and foramen magnum. This can create an obstruction to cerebrospinal fluid flow due to blockage of the fourth ventricle leading to hydrocephalus. The more severe cases are accompanied by pressure on the brainstem, creating a disturbance in the function of brainstem centers and cranial nerve deficits that may manifest themselves with difficulty in swallowing, stridor, respiratory difficulty, and even apnea. This is termed the Arnold–Chiari malformation.

Not all myelomeningoceles develop into hydrocephalus. Thus, though over 90% of infants with thoracic and lumbar myelomeningoceles develop hydrocephalus, only 40 to 45% of those at the sacral level develop this disorder. Approximately 10 to 15% of meningoceles develop into hydrocephalus. Hydrocephalus is not part of the syndrome of spinal dysrhaphia or spinal hamartomas. Thus, spinal lipomas and lipomeningoceles do not develop hydrocephalus.

CLINICAL AND MANAGEMENT IMPLICATIONS OF PATHOGENESIS

When faced with any of the spinal defects in the newborn period, the neonatologist must decide which disease he is dealing with and consequently the degree of urgency in the management of the child. Likewise, the degree of multidisciplinary support and genetic and social work counseling for the family are ascertained.

This can only be done with a thorough knowledge of the pathology and the correct support from the consulting services. It would be most inappropriate to indicate to the parents of a newborn with a spinal hamartoma that they should look forward to having a future with a child who will be paralyzed in his lower extremities, develop hydrocephalus, and require a shunt. Consequently, in all these disorders, the thorough and expeditious evaluation of the patient and diagnosis is what allows for not only immediate management when needed, but also appropriate support for the parents of this child who will be experiencing great anxiety.

No extensive test is needed whatsoever. The physical examination will determine the level of the pathology and the type of pathology. The neurological examination will determine the future outlook for the child. This, in itself, should be sufficient to diagnose the disease, institute therapy, or order other tests. Neurosurgical consultation is the primary support needed at the time.

NEONATAL DIAGNOSIS IN REFERENCE TO MANAGEMENT

Upon hearing that a child has been born with a midline defect, the neonatologist should examine the patient himself before making any decisions or counseling. The neurosurgical evaluation is immediately needed in case urgent therapy should be instituted. There is a reason behind simultaneous evaluation by a neonatologist and by a neurosurgeon. The neurosugreon will assess the local pathology, determine its characteristics, classify it, determine whether there is neurological impairment or not, and then will be able to communicate to the parents whether there is an urgent need for neurosurgical intervention, and where there is a need for it, what other tests are needed, if any. It is not uncommon for midline anomalies to be associated with other systemic mesodermal defects: cardiac anomalies, thoracic rib cage anomalies, dextrocardia, abnormal kidneys, and fused kidneys are some of the examples. Thus, if the neurological surgeon is considering early intervention and general anesthesia, the role of the neonatologist is to ascertain that there are no contraindications or related disorders that would make the urgent neurosurgical aspect of examination be deferred because of systemic or related anomalies that would contraindicate or weigh against neurosurgical therapy. It is with this team that the early appropriate management decisions can be made.

As previously related, a myelomeningocele will characteristically have no skin covering the defect, will have a neural exposure of the neural placode in varying degrees, and will have obvious denervation to varying degrees according to its level. The meningoceles, lipomeningoceles, occult spinal defects, and related disorders will be covered by skin. This simple evaluation alone already determines in the neurosurgeon's assessment whether an urgent operation is needed or whether the operation can be deferred. The reason for this relates to the outcome if the skin defect is allowed to remain following birth or if it is closed. In the untreated myelomeningocele patients of the retrospective study of Laurence, those patients that went on to die in the first few months of life expired because of bacterial infection, with a meningocerebritis and sepsis. Thus, if one is to treat the skin defect that would result in contamination, urgent repair of the area is mandate. Accordingly, this is the first stage of the neurosurgical assessment. There is another important reason to proceed this way, aside from outcome, in reference to survival. It refers to quality of outcome in those patients with myelomeningoceles, who underwent an early life infection especially from gram-negative bacteria, uniformly the intellectual outcome was worse than those who did not.

For the defects in which there is skin covering, the diagnostic tests will have to be performed prior to operative intervention (*vide infra*) to determine the underlying pathology and to guide the operative intervention. Thus, these conditions that require early intervention certainly are not urgent ones. This applies to meningoceles, lipomeningoceles, and occult spinal conditions.

In the decision-making as to whether a myelomeningocele would benefit from aggressive management, that is, early closure and subsequent shunt surgery if needed, the decision is made by the parents obviously, but the neurosurgeon and neonatologist will counsel in reference to the existing clinical state of the newborn. The presence of a small sacral myelomeningocele defect is accompanied by minimal evidence of denervation. This is because the primary innervation of the S2, S3, and S4 dermatomes relate to sphincters. Often then, the involvement of S1 dermatome is barely visible in the examination of the child and good motor function is present in the extremities. Accordingly, this child can lead a competitive, productive, and independent life because he will be fully ambulatory with or without minimal orthopedic support, with urological support, and very possibly without hydrocephalus. The counseling from the medical standpoint then would be to obviously give this newborn and the family the utmost support and encouragement for repair of the defect. Opposite such a situation is a child who is born with significant cardiac and renal anomalies, with a myelomeningocele situated at a thoracic level which then leads to an obvious finding of gross denervation of the lower extremities, and possibly with a large head already due to intrauterine hydrocephalus. Under these circumstances, the counseling given, due to the clinical state of the newborn, is to discourage treatment if that is the state of mind of the parents. Obviously as previously stated, the decision should be made by the parents, the physician and supportive personnel should relay information on the future of the child in reference to the present clinical state.

DIAGNOSTIC PROCEDURES

The primary form of diagnosis is the physical examination by a physician experienced in assessing these developmental anomalies and assessing the neurologic significance and neurologic findings. The myelomeningocele defect is, for the most part, obvious. The only diagnostic procedure the child will then need is a rapid systemic assessment for major anomalies. Thus, a chest x-ray assessment for gross cardiac abnormalities aside from the physical examination is indicated. Certainly, routine blood studies, screening coagulation studies, and urinalysis are of assistance in determining that a child is in an optimal state for urgent surgery. The CT scan of the brain is certainly not required at this point unless one suspects a neonatal presentation of a symptomatic Arnold–Chiari malformation because of stridor at rest or on crying. Crowing or respiratory difficulty should make the neonatologist suspicious. In that case, one should be aware that vocal cord paresis in varying degrees is present. Thus, extubation may not be possible if a patient is intubated for surgery. Early assessment of the vocal cords by direct examination in the operating room at the time of the myelomeningocele repair is needed.

More sophisticated studies are needed in those situations in which a meningocele is suspected to differentiate it from a lipomeningocele, which would require a different form of operative intervention, a spinal hamartoma, and the spinal teratoma. In the neonatal period, these assessments can be done by either high-resolution spinal computerized tomography (CT) or, if available, high—resolution spinal ultrasonography.

Plain Radiograms of the Spine

Plain radiograms of the spine are of assistance in determining the extent of bony involvement in the disease process, the magnitude of scoliosis or deformities, and the orthopedic outlook for the future. They do not give any significant information about the soft tissue, the neural elements, and the degree of involvement, and they certainly do not differentiate between a spinal hamartoma, lipoma, and meningocele. Therefore, they are of limited usefulness, but certainly of assistance in screening the spine.

High-Resoultion Spinal Ultrasonography

The fact that the infant's back is thin compared to older children and adults and that the ossification of the dorsal elements does not become evident until 10 to 12 months of age allows for spinal ultrasonography if a high-resolution system is available. The Division of Ultrasonography of the University of California, San Diego, has been performing such studies with a high-resolution real-time Picker Microview scanner. This system uses a 10 MHz transducer housed in a self-contained waterbath that is placed directly on the skin. The infant is placed prone for the examination and this usually takes 5 to 10 minutes. Longitudinal and transverse freeze-frame images are recorded on x-ray film by means of a multiformat camera. In addition, of importance is the fact that videotape recordings of real-time examination can be made in all cases. The depth of penetration of this system is approximately 5 cm, which allows one to see into the area of the vertebral bodies of the spine. The detail of the system is unique. Thus, the spinal cord, central canal, ventral and posterior subarachnoid space, filum terminale, as well as the dorsal elements of the spine can be identified. If masses are present, such as lipomas, they can be seen and if there are connections between the intraspinal compartment and the subcutaneous compartment, such as in the situations of lipomas in these regions, they can be ascertained. More dramatic is the visualization in real-time of the pulsations in the subarachnoid space of the spinal cord and the cauda equina following the arteriovenous pulsatile forces. This is also important in the diagnosis of tethering of the cord since pulsations are lost in real-time.

We have now visualized approximately 60 infants with spinal high-resolution ultrasonography with this system that is described, and the diagnostic reliability of such a technique is now documented.

High-Resolution Spinal Computerized Tomography

This technique is employed in infants over 10 to 12 months when the dorsal elements are ossified and the posterior elements thickened. The high-resolution spinal ultrasonography system does not permit adequate visualization of the underlying spinal structures.

The disadvantage of high-resolution spinal CT over ultrasonography is that sedation or general anesthesia is required to keep the child immobile and ionizing radiation is employed, which is not the case with ultrasonography. However, the detail of the imaging with the new systems that we employ (GE-8800, GE-9800, Somatom II and Ohio Nuclear 2020) is excellent. This technique serves as a screening and, at times, a documentary diagnostic procedure. It should be performed first without lumbar or subarachnoid contrast enhancement as this avoids the spinal puncture, the injection of contrast, and makes the procedure least invasive. Often, the diagnosis is made without the subarachnoid contrast enhancement especially used in the cases of intraspinal lipomas, lipomeningoceles, dermoid and epidermoid cysts because of the characteristics of these tissues. On the other hand, contrast is needed when a more detailed study of the nerve roots, nerve root exit zones, and subarachnoid space is needed. Sagittal midline reconstructions are of valuable assistance to the surgeon because they permit an assessment of the rostral-caudal axis of the midline in guiding the operation.

Myelography

The need for myelography is now limited; it is, at times, needed in spinal disorders of unclear anatomical level of pathology and when the subarachnoid space and nerve roots need to be studied more closely than what can be visualized on spinal CT. Myelography is less invasive when water-soluble contrast material is employed, since it is rapidly reabsorbed and thus minimizes the side effects. Myelography has a disadvantage over computerized tomography without contrast in that it requires a spinal puncture and, at times, may require more ionizing radiation. Myelography is absolutely indicated if the level of pathology is not known, since screening the whole extent of the spinal canal with computerized tomography would not be as rewarding as the myelogram and would require a large amount of ionizing radiation. Myelography is an absolute rule in many circumstances when arachnoidal bands seem to be causing the dysrhaphic condition, since it permits a clear visualization of the nerve roots. This allows for an assessment of the extent of pathology in the subarachnoid space quite clearly.

Obviously, in the neonatal period and in early infancy, spinal high-resolution ultrasonography will eliminate the need for myelography and computerized tomography in almost all cases.

EARLY MANAGEMENT OF
THE MYELOMENINGOCELE PATIENT IN
THE SPECIAL CARE NURSERY

The early phases of management are instituted after the physical diagnosis examination; later phases prepare the child for urgent neurosurgical intervention.

Following the assessment of the child to determine that there are no life-threatening systemic malformations or related problems, the appropriate preoperative blood tests and urinalysis are obtained. With myelomeningocele patients, it is commonly easy to obtain urine with the Crede maneuver due to their incontinence. It is advisable to draw a blood and urine culture, if possible, so that the results can serve as a baseline in case of sepsis or delayed referral from which sepsis has already occurred. This is important since antibiotic therapy will be instituted upon admission.

Table 2.   Elase Solution for
Topical Preparation of the
Myelomeningocele

Sterile saline solution	500 ml
Elase preparation	25000 units
Neosporin GU solution	0.5 ml

From the medical-nursing standpoint, the child should be evaluated from the point of view of ventilation, stridor or irregular respiratory rhythm. This is because in 5 to 10% of myelomeningocele patients, early symptoms of a decompensating Arnold–Chiari malformation may be present. These are sometimes thought to be due to progressive hydrocephalus, but in the first days of life the hydrocephalus is not so life-threatening due to the separation of the sutures and the compensation of the cranium by expansion *in utero*; one must remember that this hydrocephalus has been present for several months *in utero*.

Immediate topical and systemic therapy to minimize the dangers of bacterial infection of the cerebrospinal fluid pathways should be directed to the myelomeningocele. This is best done with the following regime outlined subsequently.

TOPICAL PREPARATION FOR SURGERY AND CARE OF THE MYELOMENINGOCELE

1. Place patient in prone position.
2. Place roll under patients buttocks (to elevate the buttocks and myelomeningocele, thus minimizing the contamination of the defect by urine or feces).
3. Place a sterile 4 × 4 gauze soaked in Elase solution (Table 2).
4. Measure head circumference for baseline measurements and assess respiratory pattern and ventilation for close monitoring in the preoperative status.

SYSTEMIC ANTIBIOTIC PROPHYLAXIS

Wide-spectrum antibiotic coverage is indicated. This can be performed with a synthetic penicillin and gentamycin, or related antibiotics. The therapy should be started intravenously prior to operation. The primary objective of the therapy is to obtain therapeutic levels in the cerebrospinal fluid pathways not only to prevent local wound infection and meningeal infection as well as sepsis, but also to clear the cerebrospinal fluid of bacteria for the future date of a CSF shunt placement. Thus, the institution of a foreign body in the CSF pathways will not be contaminated by bacteria that may have already penetrated.

EARLY POSTOPERATIVE MANAGEMENT OF THE MYELOMENINGOCELE PATIENT

The positioning of the patient is extremely important to minimize the risks of wound infection and wound breakdown in the area of operative repair. Since there is an underlying mesodermal defect in these patients, a natural tendency for wound dehiscence exists. Because of the proximity to the rectal structures and the local presence of urine, infection is not uncommon in the early phases of myelomeningocele postoperative repair. Thus, it becomes extremely important to have careful nursing management in this part of the postoperative care.

The patient should be prone at all times except when being picked up and held for feedings. The patient should have a roll under the buttocks to elevate the buttocks, thus keeping the myelomeningocele repair region in a higher position than the rectal and urinary sphincters to minimize pooling of urine and feces on the back wound dressing. The dressings and area of the wound should be clean at all times. To accomplish this, the patient should always be draped below the back dressing. If the dressing is subsequently removed and the wound kept uncovered, the same principles apply. Swabbing the incision two or three times daily with Betadine solution after the dressing is removed aids in minimizing bacterial contamination of the suture line. Most neurological surgeons will keep the skin sutures in for an unusually long period of time to minimize the risk of wound dehiscence.

The neurological monitoring of these postoperative myelomeningoceles is of importance. Twice daily measurements of the head circumference and assessment of the fontanelle are minimum requirements. Cerebrospinal fluid pressure can build up more quickly than in the preoperative state if there is underlying hydrocephalus, due to the fact that the back has been repaired and whatever leakage of

CSF occurred prior to the repair is now curtailed. Furthermore, the CSF pressure should not be allowed to reach high levels prior to surgical intervention with a CSF shunt procedure because the disruptive force of the CSF underneath the operative repair of the myelomeningocele can aid in back wound dehiscence. Thus, one can say that the ventriculoperitoneal shunt should be inserted when needed, not too soon and not too late, after the back wound repair. If it is too soon, the antibiotic action to clear the cerebrospinal fluid pathways of bacteria may not have been adequate, and, if it is too late, not only can progressive ventricular enlargement and additional brain damage occur, but at the same time the tendency for wound dehiscence in the myelomeningocele site and consequent infection may result. Serial cribside ultrasound examinations of the ventricular system will aid in deciding, by detecting the progressive ventriculomegaly, as to when a shunt procedure should be instituted.

Neurological observation is also needed for the early detection of decompensating Arnold-Chiari malformations. Hence, the neonatology nursing service should observe for crowing, difficulty with swallowing, pooling of secretions, and vocal cord paralysis. The first feeding is of extreme importance because that may be the point at which the paresis in swallowing and of vocal cords may be manifest for the first time; aspiration may suddenly occur with a severe apneic and, at times, irreversible insult. Should that occur, the patient should not be fed and pediatric otolaryngological consultation should be obtained to determine the degree of vocal cord paralysis to be alert for the possibility of tracheostomy, and to coordinate the care with the neurosurgeon regarding any therapy that should be promptly instituted to alleviate the symptomatology from the malformation. For instance, if progressive hydrocephalus is present, the procedure of choice is the institution of a CSF shunt to relieve the intracranial pressure which, on many occasions, will abet the symptomatology of the Arnold-Chiari malformation. If, on the other hand, this has already been done and it is wise to continue treatment, a suboccipital decompressive craniectomy is indicated to relieve the posterior fossa pressure and medullary compression.

Seizures in early life in these patients are very uncommon unless complicating factors of fluid and electrolyte balance and related problems occur.

SUBSEQUENT MANAGEMENT IN
THE SPECIAL CARE NURSERY OF THE CHILD WITH
MYELOMENINGOCELE

Subsequent to the first phases of recovery of the myelomeningocele patient, care is limited to observation, support, and determination of other complex problems. Urological and orthopedic consultations are deferred until the back wound is well healed as documented by suture removal and good apposition of wound edge. At that point the child will be moveable, he does not have to be kept in the prone position, and orthopedic manipulations and urological testing can be performed. Prior to discharge from the nursery, all of these patients should have an intravenous pyelogram, not only for a baseline study for future reference and close urological follow-up studies, but also to determine that no major developmental anomaly of the renal system or gross hydronephrosis is present that would mandate early aggressive urological intervention, such as vesicostomy or intermittent catheterization. Voiding cystourethrograms are not indicated at this early age. The studies needed primarily relate to the status of the calyceal system and observation of gross anomalies. By definition, these children have neurogenic bladder and, if reflux is present, not much is done in early life for the management of it.

Orthopedic consultation is obtained as previously indicated to determine the degree of involvement of the lower extremities, the presence of hip dysplasia, the need for any support systems for the hips and/or leg casts for the common foot deformities.

The child is then discharged and followed up in the multidisciplinary setting for the spinal defective children.

EARLY MANAGEMENT OF THE CHILD WITH
SPINA BIFIDA (SPINAL DYSRHAPHIA)

Approximately 50 percent of children with spinal dysrhaphia will manifest a cutaneous marker that may indicate underlying spinal dysrhaphism. The classical cutaneous markers for such a problem are deep dimples in the lumbar and lumbrosacral junction, local masses (such as occurs with lipomas or lipomeningoceles), an exuberant tuft of hair localized in the midline, hemangiomas of the midline, spinal aplasia cutis with or without hemangiomas and others. In other situations no cutaneous marker is visible, but obvious asymmetry and deformity of the lower extremities may be present, such as a smaller foot on one side, a pes cavus deformity, and asymmetry of the legs due to intrauterine denervation of a gastrocnemius muscle. These findings are consistent with the orthopedic syndrome described by Lassman et al. The urological syndrome of urinary tract infections and related conditions due to denervation of the bladder and sphincters does not become manifest in this early period.

Upon noting the above findings the child should be evaluated for any other systemic anomalies, as done in any newborn, but the diagnostic procedures should be geared towards spinal x-rays centered at the level of the anomaly and spinal x-rays centered to the lumbosacral spine when the findings of the orthopedic syndrome are found. Plain radiographs of those regions looking for vertebral body abnormalities, malformed sacrum, hemisacrum, sacral agenesis, and related anomalies are noticeable. On the other hand, a defect of the dorsal elements of the spine is not usually detected because of the lack of spinal ossification.

The definitive diagnostic test at this point will then be spinal high-resolution real-time ultrasonography to visualize the neural elements as previously described.

Upon confirming the presence of the anomaly, the neurosurgical consultant will then decide upon timing for elective surgery. The surgery is done early in life, but on an elective basis. All patients, prior to discharge, should have an intravenous pyelogram since associated renal anomalies may be present; baseline measurements will be needed in case neurogenic bladder develops at this time or at a future date, and the appropriate follow-up studies will then be instituted with a pediatric urology consultant.

As previously stated, early life surgery is indicated to minimize the progressive and insidious neurological damage that occurs with development which is irreversible. Operative intervention is performed via microneurosurgery and laser surgery to minimize damage to the surrounding nerve structures that are normal, thus assuring, by the technique minimal risk of creating neurological problems not present beforehand. Rectal electromyographic monitoring permits surgery to be carried out in the cauda equina or in the conus, as monitoring of the dermatomes relates to bladder sphincter and rectal sphincter function.

CONCLUSIONS

The early life prompt assessment of spinal disorders, such as myelomeningocele and spinal dysrhaphia, is of extreme importance to obtaining good quality outcome, reduction in the incidence of complications, and aid in the early and definitive management of these diseases. Therefore, thorough knowledge of the topic by the neonatologist and neonatal nursing staff will assure not only early detection of the disorder and the institution of the appropriate and immediate steps to aid in neurosurgical evaluation and correction, but also will minimize unnecessary procedures and will promote good quality outcome following the discharge from the special care nursery.

REFERENCES

1. Ames, M.D., and Schut, L. Results of Treatment of 171 Consecutive Myelo-meningoceles—1963 to 1976. *Pediatrics 50*:466-470, 1972.
2. James, H.E., and Walsh, J.W. Spinal Dysrhaphism. *Current Problems in Pediatrics, 8*, 1981.
3. James, H.E., and Oliff, M. Computer Tomography in Spinal Dysrhaphism. *J. Comput. Assist. Tomogr. 1*:391-397, 1977.

CHAPTER 8

Apnea and Hypoventilation in Infancy

Daniel C. Shannon, M.D.

DEFINITIONS

From inspection of breathing patterns recorded for 12 hours at monthly intervals on 100 infants, we determined that the longest episode of normal apnea, almost invariably following a sigh, was 14 sec. Therefore, we define abnormal apnea as an episode of 15 sec. or greater.

Hypoventilation occurs when the total alveolar ventilation per minute is insufficient to clear metabolically produced CO_2; thus, by definition, it is a rise in P_{CO_2} in alveolar gas and, therefore, in arterial blood. Because these two pressures are in ready equilibrium across the alveolar-capillary membrane, measurement of either is sufficient to define alveolar ventilation. Alveolar P_{CO_2} can simply be measured by sampling exhaled air at nose or mouth in which the last part of the breath came from alveoli. The level of ventilation varies with state and is most easily measured during quiet sleep when defects in control of breathing are generally more evident. Hypoventilation can occur either because of inadequate tidal volume or frequency, generally the former. It is difficult to diagnose by observation because we cannot visually recognize any but major reduction in tidal volume. For example, with a normal breath the chest diameter changes about 0.5 cm in the newborn; at a half normal tidal volume,

Perinatal Neurology and Neurosurgery. Edited by R. A. Thompson, J. R. Green, and S. D. Johnsen. Copyright © 1985 by Spectrum Publications, Inc.

the change is 0.24 cm. Therefore, we first recognize hypoventilation from its consequences and confirm its presence by measuring P_{CO_2}.

CONSEQUENCES

The consequences of apnea and hypoventilation are similar, differing only in their time course. The first effects are a decrease in alveolar P_{O_2} and an increase in P_{CO_2}, which then are reflected in blood leaving the lung and thus in areterial blood. The rate of change in O_2 and CO_2 over time depends on the amount of gas stored in lung and tissue especially compared to the metabolic rate, that is, the rate of O_2 consumption. The time limit of tolerance depends, in addition, on hemoglobin concentration and on the redistribution of cardiac output to vital organs. T = Vol. O_2 stored/vol. O_2 consumed per minute. It is no surprise then that symptoms and adverse consequences are seen in the two systems most critically dependent on O_2 delivery, that is, the cardiovascular and central nervous system.

In the cardiovascular system, hypoxia and hypercapnia have several effects both immediate and delayed. In the pulmonary circulation, alveolar hypoxia ($PA_{O_2} < 65$ mm Hg) cause vasoconstriction increasing right ventricular afterload. In the cerebral and coronary circulation, hypoxemia as well as hypercapnia bring instant vasodilation via autoregulation. Hypercapnia, in particular, immediately increases catecholamine output from the adrenal medulla. The net early effect is an increase in blood flow to heart and brain and an increased right and left ventricular afterload. Hypercapnia through cerebral vasodilation and increased CSF production raises CSF pressure. Failure to meet aerobic energy requirements and increased perfusion pressure particularly in tenuous periventricular neonatal vessels are thought to contribute to cerebral damage and its consequences—seizure, spastic diplegia, and developmental retardation. Repeated episodes may not only compound these adverse effects but also promote increased muscularity in the pulmonary circulation. This will further increase RV afterload and, with each successive episode, limit LV output thus establishing a self-reinforcing positive feedback loop favoring more severe hypoxia.

These events probably explain the occurrence of brain damage as well as the pulmonary and systemic hypertension that may precipitate cardiac failure in more severely affected patients.

The rapidity of change in arterial P_{O_2} and P_{CO_2} with apnea is not often appreciated. We have found that measured changes are

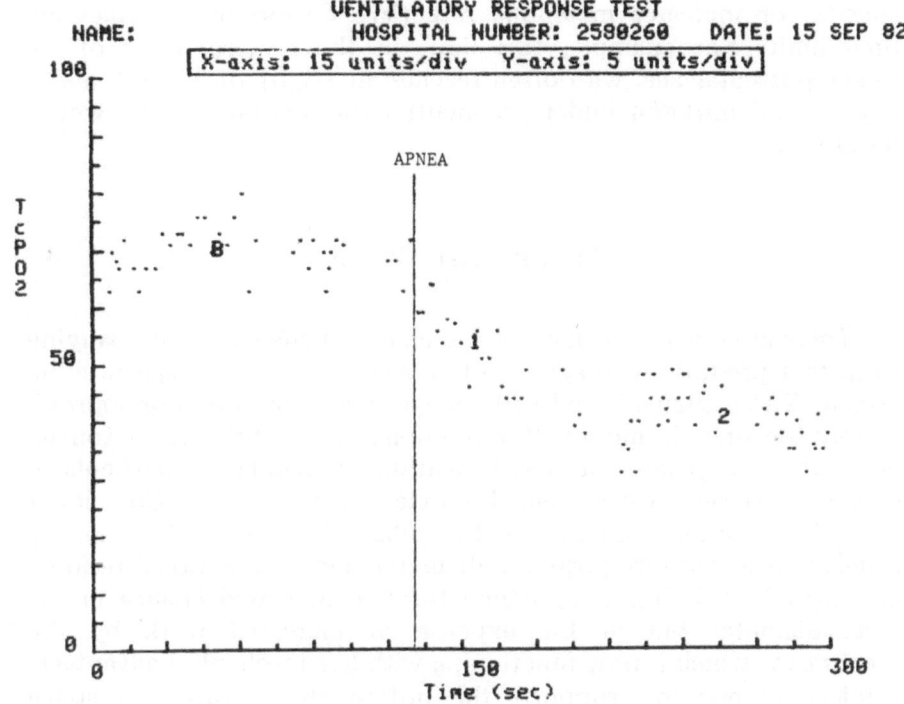

Figure 1. Change in P_{O_2} over time during apnea P_{O_2} reached 30 mm Hg after 75 sec.

comparable to those that can be predicted. Using the parameters that determine O_2 stores in lung and circulation compared to those that affect O_2 consumption rate, I have calculated that PA_{O_2} in arterial blood would decrease from 90 to 25 mm Hg in 65 sec. Figure 1 shows the measured fall typically observed in an infant. An arterial P_{O_2} of 25 mm Hg approximates the P_{50}, the level at which hemoglobin is 50% saturated. Using the observation that normal infants can be apneic for 14 sec. and that under the best of circumstances PA_{O_2} reaches the P_{50} after 45 sec. of apnea, one can estimate the duration of permissible apnea in a given infant beyond which an alarm should sound alerting medical staff or parents to an at-risk condition. In practice, we generally use a 20 sec. delay and caution caretakers to observe for color change before intervening because most episodes of abnormal apnea will end spontaneously and are not known to produce measurable hypoxic injury. Note that any factor which reduces stores (low lung volume, hypoxemia or anemia) or increases metabolic rate (V_{O_2}) shortens the tolerable time limit. For example, this limit in the preterm baby of six weeks postnatal age, who often reaches an [Hgb] of 7 gm/dl and a V_{O_2} of 15 ml/kg/m under non-neutral thermal conditions, would be 11 sec.

SLEEP AND APNEA

There are several mechanical and chemical changes accompanying sleep that predispose to apnea or hypoventilation and exaggerate the effects. These changes tend to be magnified in infants. For approximately the first six months, the hypopharynx is shallow, the tongue abuts the soft palate, and nasal breathing is mandatory particularly during active sleep when skeletal muscle tone is inhibited. Coincident inhibition of intercostal muscles destabilizes the chest wall promoting a decrease in anterior-posterior diameter and in functional residual capacity. Ventilation is sustained through increased change in the axial diameter but at the expense of increased work by the diaphragm, which is now functioning with less mechanical advantage. Clinical observation supports the notion that obstructive apnea develops in infants when these anatomical and functional characteristics are compounded by further obstruction such as neck flexion in the preterm baby or an upper respiratory infection in the infant.

Apnea or hypoventilation can be prolonged in quiet sleep when alveolar ventilation is determined mainly by the chemical controllers. Patients who lack a medullary H^+ ion controller characteristically breathe normally when awake and hypoventilate mildly in active sleep and profoundly in quiet sleep.

Gas exchange is more severely perturbed in the sleeping infant than in the child or adult; oxygen stores are less and O_2 consumption rate is greater. During active sleep, functional residual capacity, the lung volume at end expiration, is vulnerable because inactive intercostal muscles fail to oppose the elastic recoil of the lung which then empties rapidly into the atmosphere. Hemoglobin concentration is relatively low especially around six weeks thus reducing carrying capacity for O_2. It is not unusual for the infant born preterm to reach a hemoglobin concentration of 7 gm/dl at this time. Finally, metabolic rate is two- to three-fold higher in the infant. The net effect is that critical oxygen levels will be reached in the infant in one-fourth to one-eighth the time seen in the child or adult.

Termination of apnea during sleep is at least partly dependent on arousal to a state in which skeletal muscle control of respiratory muscles is more active. It has been proposed, based on experimental data, that the arousal thresholds, particularly to hypoxia, are lower in infants prone to prolonged apnea. The neurochemical basis for arousal should provide a fruitful area of investigation.

CLINICAL APNEA SYNDROMES

In order to provide a logical framework for the clinician, I have divided apnea into those episodes that occur silently compared to those associated with prior or subsequent noisy breathing. The basis for this division is that infants with noisy breathing tend to have an anatomical basis for obstructive apnea. A further useful division is the presence or absence of neurological signs of disease. This excludes signs that can result from hypoxia or hypercapnia alone. Next, I have found it useful both when documenting the history and when considering a diagnostic evaluation to enumerate the cardinal categories of disease. Beyond this the following diagrams (Tables 1-6) are self-explanatory.

Table 1.

Apnea

Silent — (Probably abnormal control of muscles regulating Δ lung volume)

Noisy — Probably abnormality affecting airway patency

Silent branch:
- Neurological signs (+): Infections, Congenital, Toxic-Metabolic, Neoplastic
- Neurological signs (−): Metabolic, Idiopathic

Noisy branch:
- Structural (+): Neurological signs (+) (−)
- Structural (−): Neurological signs (+) (−)

Table 2. Apnea—Silent with Neurological Signs

Infectious

   Brain stem meningoencephalitis

Trauma

   At birth
   Surgical

Developmental defect

   Myelomeningocele
   Brainstem malformation, for example, Mohr's syndrome
   Syringomyelia

Toxic-metabolic

   Opiates and depressants, psychotropics, phenothiazines
   Leigh's encephalopathy
   Inborn errors—organic acidemias, urea cycle
   Congenital central hypoventilation
   Hyperthermia
   Hypothyroid
   Botulism

Neoplastic

   Brainstem tumor
   Tumor with intracranial hypertension

Degenerative

   Multiple Sclerosis

We will now examine in detail two apnea syndromes, the apnea/hypoventilation syndrome associated with Sudden Infant Death (SIDS) and the obstructive apnea that accompanies partial upper airway obstruction.

HYPOVENTILATION SYNDROME

Although the central hypoventilation syndrome has been described in less than 50 infants, the diagnosis is being made with increasing frequency in neonatal intensive care units and physicians need guidance in recommending and providing treatment. In addition, we and others have identified a larger group of infants who manifest hypoventilation and defective ventilatory response to

**Table 3. Apnea—Silent without
Neurological Signs**

Infectious

    Airway infection especially RSV
    Brain stem encephalitis

Trauma

    Late complication CSF leak
    Induced

Developmental defect

    Gastroesophageal reflex
    Absent corpus callosum

Toxic-metabolic

    Seizure
    Idiopathic

**Table 4. Apnea—Noisy Breathing with
Structural Defect**

Neurological signs

    Gastroesophageal reflux
    Abductor cord paralysis

No neurological signs

    Infectious

        Urinary in young infant
        Tonsillar and adenoid hypertrophy
        Diphtheria

    Developmental defect

        Noise to carina

    Foreign body

    Neoplasia

Table 5. Apnea—Noisy Breathing without Structural Defect

Neurological signs

Moebius

No neurological signs

Idiopathic

CO_2 in association with near-SIDS episodes. Most near SIDS infants, however, do not have this defect in chemical regulation.

In order to confirm the diagnosis, we measure ventilation using a pneumotachygraph connected to the endotracheal or tracheostomy tube adaptor or to nasal prongs. The voltage signal generated from a differential pressure transducer, which is linear with pressure difference, is integrated with time to yield sequential tidal volumes. A fraction of expired air (about 60 ml/min) is sampled continuously from a sidehole in the tubed adaptor and drawn through an infrared CO_2 analyzer. After phase alignment of these signals, they are digitized at 100 Hz and stored on computer tape. The variables of interest are displayed and instantaneous ventilation as a function of time or partial pressure of gases is calculated. State is assessed by a standard method. Inspired gas is altered by providing 4 to 5% CO_2 in the air, 15% O_2 or 100% O_2 to the awake infant and the ventilatory responses are recorded.

Unless the patient has experienced chronic hypoventilation with consequent elevation of bicarbonate, ventilation and blood gas values, while awake, are normal.

Table 6. Six-Hour Sleep Study

Stage[a]	1	2
%	33	67
P_{O_2}	48–81	48–70
P_{CO_2}	40–52	42–50
Apnea (10–15 sec.)		
Central syndrome	4	1
Obstructive syndrome	5	

[a]No stage 3, 4 or REM.

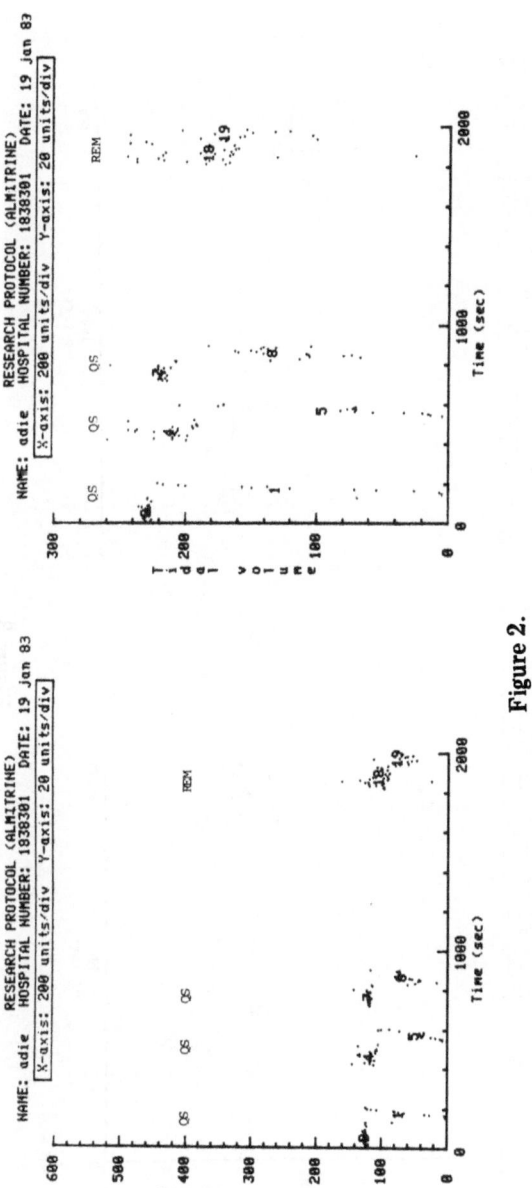

Figure 2.

Daniel C. Shannon

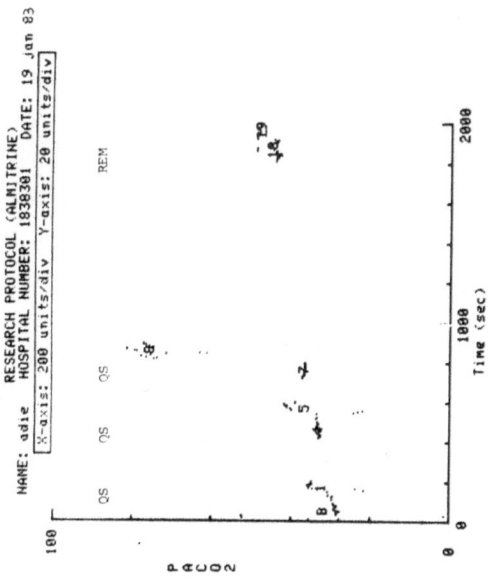

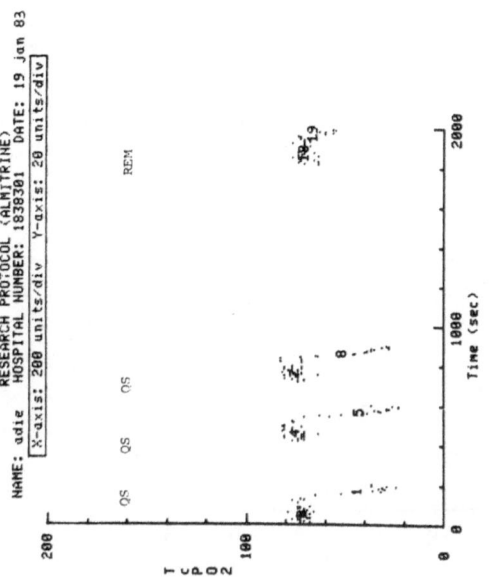

Figure 3.

Ventilation in REM sleep is normal or mildly reduced and in quiet sleep is even more reduced. Tidal volumes are reduced (Figure 2) while frequency is preserved and results in PA_{CO_2} values over 46 mm Hg (Figure 3). In patients with more marked degree, the PA_{CO_2} can rise over 100 mm Hg. We have found that during wakefulness the ventilatory responses to altered inspired gas are similar from one patient to the next; the response to 4 to 50% CO_2 in air breathing exhibited a blunted or even negative slope (Figure 4), the response to 15% O_2 was variable and improved with age; in infancy, it may be followed by ventilatory depression and obvious cynanosis; the response to 100% O_2 was characterized by ventilatory depression to as little as 63% of resting levels.

Beyond four months of age, V_A during quiet sleep was improved so that PA_{CO_2} seldom exceeded 67 mm Hg. Without a tracheostomy tube in place, it is difficult to repeat measurements beyond six months of age. However, in those with more marked hypoventilation in infancy, improvement with age is rare.

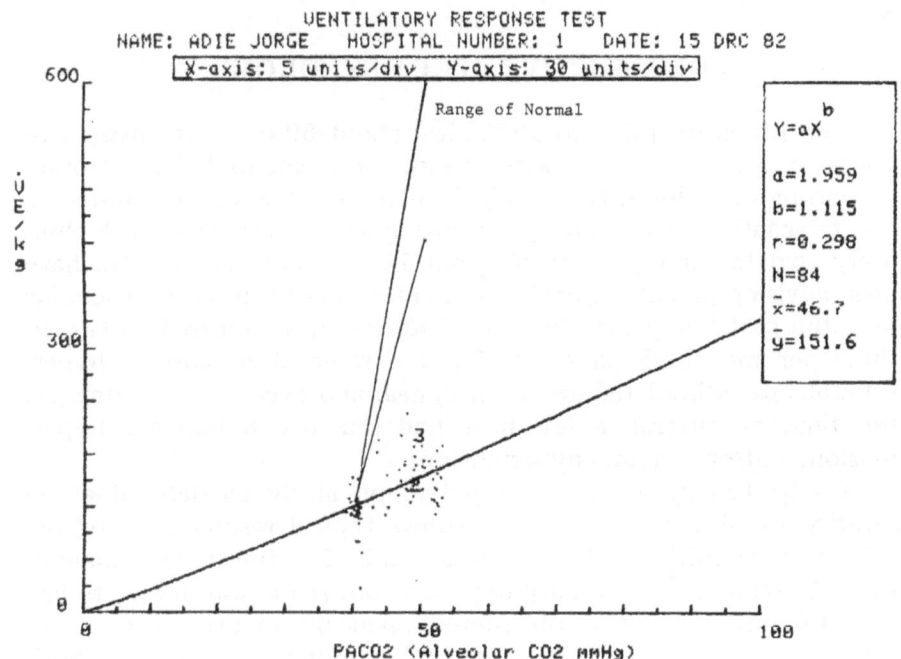

Figure 4.

In addition to the defect in chemical regulation of the ventilatory pump, there is also a defect in regulation of upper airway muscles with a tendency to manifest paradoxical chest wall movement in quiet sleep (QS).

Those with subtle degrees of hypoventilation (PA_{CO_2} 55 mm Hg in QS) can be safely managed with cardiorespiratory monitor at home and often benefit from treatment with methylxanthines. The rest require support of ventilation by a mechanical respirator or by phrenic nerve pacing.

Seizures and delayed gross motor development are common in infancy but are rare beyond six years of age. In a few cases, aganglionosis of the GI tract and tumors of neural crest origin bave been described.

Biventricular cardiac failure develops in these infants if alveolar hypoxia and hypercapnia persist either because of inadequate spontaneous or inadequate mechanical ventilation. This in turn can affect neurological development. Cardiac failure resolves usually within one week after minute ventilation is increased by mechanical or chemical means.

OBSTRUCTIVE APNEA SYNDROME

The literature prior to 1975 cites about 50 cases of obstructive sleep apnea associated with tonsil and adenoid hypertrophy presenting in children two to eight years of age with cor pulmonale and retardation. From a busy consulting service, I saw one such child every two to three years until about 1978. Since pediatricians have been advising parents against routine removal of tonsils and adenoids over the past five years, the rate of referral has increased to two to three per month. Most cases now are referred because of hypersomnolence, school failure, sleep apnea, and excessive sweating. At the time of referral, a few have had seizures, pulmonary hypertension, and/or systemic hypertension.

I rely heavily on a sleep polygraph study to determine the severity of obstruction. Table 6 shows typical results. Any of the following conditions should be grounds for tonsil and adenoid (T & A) removal: pulmonary hypertension, reduction in P_{O_2} to less than 60 mm Hg during obstructed breathing or average P_{CO_2} in excess of 45 mm Hg. Apneic episodes in these patients are both obstructive and central. Persistence of central apnea or hypoventilation after T & A removal suggests that a defect in control of respiratory muscles may explain the occurrence of inadequate gas exchange in some children and not others even though the degree of obstruction appears to be similar. A lateral neck radiograph especially during sleep is very helpful in suggesting an anatomical cause of obstruction.

Both tonsils and adenoids should be removed. Because of the precarious circulatory status of these children, the first postoperative day should be in an intensive care unit equipped to deal with the difficult airway. In a few patients, removal of T & A for obstructive sleep apnea in the first 18 months has been followed by regrowth of tissue and need for repeat surgery.

The consequence of other lesions that compromise pulmonary gas exchange are similar to those that accompany central hypoventilation or obstructive sleep apnea. Likewise, the indications for treatment and the methods of support are similar.

CHAPTER 9

Clinical Neurological Assessment of the Neonate

Alfred W. Brann, Jr., M.D.

INTRODUCTION

As a result of increased knowledge in neonatal-perinatal medicine, there has been a progressive reduction in the neonatal mortality rate in the last 30 years. In the United States as a whole, the neonatal mortality rate has been reduced from 12.3/1000 live births in 1974 to 9.9/1000 live births in 1977. Although the United States ranks 16th in the world with respect to the neonatal mortality rate, it has the lowest birthweight-specific neonatal mortality rate in the world.

In concert with a decrease in the neonatal mortality rate, the incidence of long-term neurological sequelae in children who have been high-risk neonates has been reduced over the last 30 years. Neurological and developmental handicaps in the surviving preterm infants born before 1960 ranged from 60 to 70%, whereas current central nervous system (CNS) morbidity ranges from 10 to 30%.. The various types of CNS sequelae detected in surviving children who have been high-risk neonates include the following:

A. Motor deficits
 1. Spastic diplegia
 2. Spastic quadriplegia
 3. Spastic hemiplegia
 4. Choreoathetosis

Perinatal Neurology and Neurosurgery. Edited by R. A. Thompson, J. R. Green, and S. D. Johnsen. Copyright © 1985 by Spectrum Publications, Inc.

B. Mental retardation
C. Disorders of abstract reasoning
D. Seizures
E. Sensory abnormalities
   1. Hearing deficits
   2. Visual abnormalities
      a. Retrolental fibroplasia
      b. Eye motility dysfunction
F. Posthemorrhagic hydrocephalus
G. Microcephaly.

The perinatally related etiologies of the above mentioned types of central nervous system sequelae seen in high-risk neonates are quite varied and include the following:

Chromosomal abnormalities
Dysmorphic syndromes
Environmental agents
Malnutrition
Infections
Trauma
Intracranial hemorrhage
Inherited metabolic diseases
Metabolic disorders
   Hypoxic ischemia
   Hypoglycemia
   Hyperbilirubinemia
   Hypernatremia.

In considering the general reduction in the incidence of central nervous system sequelae, there has not been a uniform reduction in the incidence of handicapped children from each of these etiologies. From hospital-based data from the U.S. as well as from population-based data from Sweden, the recent reduction in the incidence of neurologically handicapped children has primarily been related to a reduction in cerebral diplegia especially in surviving low-birthweight infants. This would fall primarily in the category of hypoxic ischemia. It is important to recognize that Downs Syndrome and meningomyelocele, two conditions in the categories of chromosomal abnormalities and dysmorphic syndromes, account for more children with CNS dysfunction than from other etiologies. A second major point to recognize is that, although there has been major success in reducing the incidence of CNS sequallae in children who were preterm infants with a reduction in cerebral diplegia, there are actually more children with cerebral palsy who were full-term infants than who were preterm infants. This relates to the fact that, although the incidence of cerebral palsy is approximately 90/1,000 live born preterm infants vs. 3.38/1,000 in live born full-term infants, most of the births in this country, 93%, are full-term infants.

One of the factors in the reduction of the incidence in CNS morbidity in surviving children who are high-risk neonates is an increase in the ability to accurately assess the nervous system in the neonate. With the advent of more effective and accurate noninvasive diagnostic tools such as computed axial tomography, ultrasonography, intracranial pressure monitoring, and Doppler measurements of cerebral blood flow velocity, more refined clinical neuropathological correlations have permitted a validation of the clinical neonatal neurological exam. Thus a more refined clinical neonatal neurological assessment as outlined below has evolved and has permitted the physician to detect neurological dysfunction; to diagnose, treat, and/or prevent specific neurological disorders; and to identify neonates at increased risks for later neurological dysfunction.

A. History
    1. Parental history
    2. Obstetric history
        a. Past pregnancy outcome
        b. Present obstetric history
            (1) Prenatal
            (2) Intrapartum
        c. Neonatal history
B. General pediatric examination
    1. Gestational age
    2. Head size and shape
    3. Cranial sutures
    4. Fontanels
    5. Transillumination of skull
    6. Bruit
    7. Facies
    8. Minor anomalies
    9. Eye
    10. Hepatosplenomegaly
    11. Skin lesions
    12. Back

      13. Odor
      14. Contractures
   C. Neurological examination
       1. Level of consciousness
       2. Motor system
         a. Posture
         b. Tone
         c. Strength
         d. Movements
       3. Reflexes
       4. Sensory system
       5. Cranial nerve tests
         a. Fix and follow: II, III, IV, VI, Cortex
         b. Pupillary response: II, III
         c. Doll's eye: III, IV, VI, medial longitudinal fasciculus, VIII
         d. Suck: V, VII, XII
         e. Swallow: IX, X
         f. Hearing: VIII
   D. Interpretation
         a. Low risk
         b. High risk
         c. Suspect.

The optimum neonatal clinical neurological assessment as outlined above includes more than just the neurological examination. The general mechanics of performing this assessment are explained in the following sections entitled: history, general pediatric examination, and neurological examination.

HISTORY

A detailed account of the parental, obstetric, and neonatal histories is necessary for a systematic evaluation of the neonatal nervous system. The parental history should include the age and race of both parents, familial disease in both parents' families and the mother's past medical history.

A complete obstetric history should include information regarding the present pregnancy and details of all previous pregnancies and their outcomes. The present obstetric history should include details of both the prenatal and intrapartum course, with complete information regarding any bleeding, infections during pregnancy, or maternal drug exposure.

The neonatal history should include information regarding the delivery room course and the subsequent nursery course. Knowledge of the Apgar score at 1, 5, 10, 15, and 20 minutes along with information about methods of resuscitation in the delivery room is of particular note and is essential. Infants who have Apgar scores of 7 to 10 have been found to be at very low risk for an abnormal transition to extrauterine life and for later abnormal neurological development. Data now show that a significantly low Apgar score is a score of 0-3. The level of 0-3 is a "significantly low score" because of the higher mortality and CNS morbidity in infants with this score than with either a 4-6 or a 7-10 score. The longer the score is low, the greater is its significance. An infant with a 0-3 Apgar score at one minute has a mortality of some 5 to 10% which rises to approximately 53% if that Apgar score is maintained for 20 minutes. In surviving full-term neonates with an Apgar score of 0-3 at five minutes, the incidence of cerebral palsy was approximately 1%. If this Apgar score was sustained for 15 minutes the percent of survivors having cerebral palsy was 9% with a dramatic rise to 57% for infants who sustained an Apgar of 0-3 for 20 minutes. There was not a significant difference in the incidence of CNS morbidity and mortality between infants who had an Apgar score of 4-6 and 7-10.

Although a low Apgar score is known to be bad, a low score does not imply any specific etiology. It can be due to any one of the following six major causes: asphyxia, drugs, hypovolemia, trauma, infection, and/or anomalies. For instance, in ascribing a low Apgar score to asphyxia, one should have positive signs of intrapartum asphyxia, while also ruling out the other five causes of low Apgar score.

The neonatal history from the nursery course should include detailed information regarding particular relevant clinical events such as seizures, cyanotic spells, apneic episodes, diminished or absent crying, distinct and/or prolonged episodes of hypotonia, decreased activity, poor suck, and prolonged requirement of gavage feedings. The length and severity of biochemical and physiological variables such as hypoglycemia, hyperbilirubinemia, hypoxemia, and shock during a neonate's course should be documented because their presence could be important in identifying the child who may be at risk for subsequent abnormal development and/or who requires special follow-up care.

GENERAL PEDIATRIC EXAMINATION

There are particular findings in the general pediatric examination that are of special importance from the neurological standpoint. The head should be examined for size, shape, status of anterior fontanel, and evidence of any trauma such as cephalohematoma or fractures. Cranial bruits should be noted, especially in a newborn with congestive heart failure in the first 24 hours of life. Peculiar facies, associated with over 300 specific syndromes and/or other designated minor anomalies, should be identified since the central nervous system frequently is involved with a generalized malformation. If three or more minor anomalies are identified, the chances of a major internal anomaly occurring is approximately 90%. The examination of the eyes is described under the examination of cranial nerve II. Of particular importance from the neurological standpoint is evidence of skin lesions, such as the vesicles of congenital herpes, petechiae, cutaneous lesions of other TORCH agents, hemangioma of Sturge-Weber disease, pigmented lesions of neurofibromatosis, the pale nevi of tuberous sclerosis, or the vesicles of incontinentia pigmenti. Hepatosplenomegaly may occur in diseases that also involve the nervous system, such as encephalitis secondary to infection with one of the TORCH agents. Abnormalities of the back should be identified, including the finding of a small dermal sinus or tuft of hair, which may indicate either a direct channel to the subarachnoid space from the skin or a significant abnormality of the lumbosacral spinal column. Abnormalities in hair texture and presence of swirls may be associated with underlying neurological disorders. The particular smell of a neonate or his urine may lead to suspicion of an aminoaciduria. The location and extent of joint contracture at birth, known specifically as arthrogryposis multiplex congenita, indicates a syndrome that is usually secondary to disease of the nervous system at some level. In some patients it may be secondary to primary joint disease.

NEUROLOGIC EXAMINATION

Introduction

Since the functional state of the neonatal nervous system is influenced by both endogenous and exogenous factors unrelated to a specific disease, these factors must be considered if an accurate neurological assessment is to be obtained. The endogenous factors primarily relate to the developmental status of the nervous system, which is dependent on gestational age and not on chronological age of the infant. Some of the pertinent endogenous/developmental factors influencing the specific level of neurological function or dysfunction are discussed in the following paragraphs.

The nervous system is a heterogeneous organ with differing regional rates of growth and development. Differentiation and development of the brain are continuing at the time of birth. Myelination shows striking regional differences in rates of development and is still far from complete at 40 weeks of gestation. It is much more advanced in the temporal lobes, midbrain, brainstem, spinal cord, and peripheral nerves than in the cerebral hemispheres. In the term neonate, dendritic sprouting and arborization are in a phase of major growth with the ongoing formation of interneuronal excitatory synaptic connections. The inhibitory synaptic connections are more numerous at this time than the excitatory ones.

An active cellular area of brain located alongside of the ventricular system is the very vascular germinal matrix composed of pleuropotential cells which differentiate and migrate out from this region to populate the cerebral hemispheres including the six layers of cortex. By 18 to 20 weeks of gestation, the developing fetus has most of its neurons. After this time, reabsorption of this vascular germinal area begins and is usually complete by 35 to 36 weeks of gestation. Until resorption of the germinal matrix, this periventricular area remains highly vascularized but with poor tissue support for the remaining vessels. This lack of tissue support may be one of the factors contributing to the occurrence of subependymal and intraventricular hemorrhage in the preterm infant.

The brain capillaries are unique because of the presence of tight junctions, decreased numbers of pinocytotic vesicles, specific plasma membrane carriers, increased numbers of mitochondria, which can oxidize several different fuels producing large amounts of ATP, and a tough basement membrane for protection during various types of stress. The basement membrane from isolated capillaries of developing animal brain is one-fourth of the thickness of that from capillaries of an adult brain. A possible reduced amount of capillary basement membrane in the preterm infant may be another factor contributing to the occurrence of subependymal and intraventricular hemorrhage.

The physiology of neuronal membranes in the newborn indicates that the neuronal pumps are less efficient and the cell membranes are more leaky than later in development. Cerebral metabolism of the newborn differs from that of the older child. The newborn is far more resistant to anoxia than is the older infant and seems better able to use both ketone bodies and anerobic glycolysis as energy sources.

Since subcortical structures of the nervous system are at a higher state of development both morphologically and neurophysiologically than cortical structures, information derived from the neonatal neurological examination reflects primarily the functional status of subcortical structures. There is, however, increasing evidence of the neonate's cortical function as manifested by rudimentary learning ability and ability to integrate sensory stimuli.

There are three exogenous factors that must be considered in the accurate assessment of the nervous system. The first factor is the time of the exam in relationship to feeding. An infant examined in the immediate postprandial state is usually sleepy with decreased responsiveness and may be hypotonic as well as hyporeflexic. That same infant examined just before feeding time may be crying, irritable, hypertonic, hyperreflexic, and jittery. The optimum time to examine an infant in relation to feedings is approximately one to two hours afterward. A second major factor that can affect the functional state of the neonate's nervous system is the ambient temperature of the examining room and/or the temperature of the neonate. Hypothermia can cause depression, and hyperthermia can result in irritability, so the infant is best examined at thermal neutrality. The third factor that can influence the findings of the neurological examination is the degree of illness of the infant. In severely ill neonates, there can be a generalized depression of the nervous system. In addition, there may be limitations on examining sick infants when they are in incubators, when they are being mechanically ventilated, and/or when they are connected to multiple monitors with several catheters in place. One must be willing to examine and reexamine a neonate to confirm the presence of significant abnormalities.

Level of Consciousness

An altered state of consciousness is a major sign of neonatal neurological impairment. The sleep and awake states of a neonate can markedly affect the functional state of a normal neonate's nervous system. It is important to ascertain the neonate's state of arousal. The neonate is best examined in the quiet alert state.

The level of consciousness is determined by an evaluation of the amount of spontaneous activity and the response to stimulation. The neonate's level of consciousness can be divided into five levels ranging from normal to abnormal. The neonate is said to be normal when in the quiet alert state, his arms and legs flexed and exhibiting symmetrical spontaneous activity that is nonstereotyped. The second level is the hyperalert state, identified in a neonate who does not sleep for extended periods of time during the first 24 hours. The eyes are wide open, possibly with a decreased blinking response as well as a decreased ability to fixate and follow. Although the activity level may be normal or decreased, it may appear increased because of the decreased threshold to all types of tactile, auditory, visual, and proprioceptive stimuli. The third level is lethargy, which can be of variable degree. There is a decrease in spontaneous activity, although the threshold for responsiveness may be decreased as just mentioned. Even though responses are delayed, there is a complete repertoire of responses to stimulation. The fourth level is stupor, where the infant's responses are limited to withdrawal of an extremity or decerebrate posturing in response only to strong noxious stimuli. Corneal and gag reflexes are absent, and respiratory rhythm may be abnormal. The fifth level is coma, with no response to external stimuli. In the neonate this is a relatively rare state, since the spinal withdrawal reflexes are almost never abolished. This state may be observed in infants on respirators who have had severe intraventricular hemorrhage.

Motor System

Posture Observation of posture should be performed both before and after removing the neonate from the crib or incubator and undressing him. Even if the neonate cannot be moved, such as when on a ventilator, much can be gained from observation of posture. When evaluating posture, it is imperative to recognize the changes that occur with gestational age. With increasing age, the infant's extremities normally begin to assume a much more flexed position.

Abnormalities of posture at rest include asymmetry between sides, as seen in the infant with a brachial plexus lesion; asymmetries between arms and legs, as seen with a spinal cord lesion; the frog-leg position with hips completely abducted and knees flexed, following severe asphyxia with severe systemic disease or with neuromuscular disease producing hypotonia or paralysis; head retraction and extensor posturing, which may occur with intracranial hemorrhage, hypoxic-ischemic encephalopathy, or meningitis. The cortical thumb (a closed hand with the thumb inside the fingers) can be a normal position of the hand in the neonate. This position is, however, not obligatory, and the neonate will periodically open the hand and extend the thumb. An obligatory cortical thumb is an early sign of cortical spinal tract dysfunction in the infant.

Tone   Muscle tone can be assessed by using the same maneuvers used in the gestational age assessment of the Dubowitz examination, including arm and leg recoil, popliteal angle, wrist-arm angle, foot dorsiflexion, hip flexion, shoulder abduction (scarf sign), head lag, and position in ventral suspension. The examiner must consider the gestational age of the infant when attempting to determine whether the tone is reduced, normal, or increased. A neonate with poor head control may, for example, be considered normal if he is a preterm infant rather than a small-for-gestational-age term infant.

The baby of 40 to 42 weeks, when in ventral suspension, should dorsiflex his back with some elevation of his head; his feet and legs remain flexed. Hypotonia, weakness, or cerebral depression may produce a baby who looks like a limp dishrag. Upright suspension with the baby supported by the examiner's hands under his arm provides good estimation of both tone and strength in the shoulder girdle, since an infant with decreased tone or strength can slip through the examiner's hands. Tone can also be assessed by movement of individual joints.

Although tone is only one of the five areas assessed in assigning the Apgar score, it has extremely important predictive value. When a low score occurs, the order of loss of the five areas is: Color, respirations, tone, reflexes, and heart rate. Following effective resuscitation, these functions reappear in the following order: Heart rate, reflexes, color, respirations, and tone. The length of time it takes for the return of tone is felt to be an indicator of the severity of the insult to the central nervous system. A delay in return of tone, if greater than two hours in the presence of signs of intrapartum asphyxia, is associated with an increased incidence of hypoxic ischemic encephalopathy in the neonate as well as significant neurological sequelae in surviving neonates.

Strength   Strength and weakness are related to the state of alertness, to gestational age, and/or to problems in the central or peripheral nervous system as well as in the muscles. Testing muscle strength is difficult in a newborn infant, and differentiating between muscle weakness and hypotonia may be impossible, since neonates who are weak are usually hypotonic or floppy. However, an adequate screening test of strength in the upper extremities and neck may be accomplished through the use of the neonate's grasp. The examiner's finger is inserted into the lateral aspect of the neonate's hand. In association with this grasp, the normal newborn should be sufficiently strong to partially support his weight as he is lifted from the supine to the sitting position. As the neonate is pulled up, the observer should feel contractions in the biceps and the shoulder girdle along with some contraction in the sternocleidomastoid muscles, preventing the head from completely falling back. Strength in the lower extremities can be assessed by observing the supporting response, the ability of the newborn to support his weight when his feet are placed on the examining table. Stepping, placing and exhibiting the crossed extensor reflexes also may be used to assess strength; asymmetries of strength should be noted.

Observations of the quality of spontaneous movements and movements that can be elicited in response to pinprick stimulation can give considerable information about strength of specific muscle groups. This information is important in localizing the level of a lesion of the spinal cord.

Movements Observation of an infant prior to being touched may reveal a variety of movements. The quantity of spontaneous movement can vary from normal to excessive to decreased. The pattern of movement observed in a normal infant during spontaneous activity can be characterized as random, symmetrical, non-stereotyped movements involving all extremities.

In addition to patterned movements, the neonate may have movements that are characterized as being either tremors, jitteriness, or seizures. Since neonatal seizures are usually caused by treatable conditions which, if left untreated, cause brain damage, it is important to identify and differentiate an infant with this type of activity from an infant who may simply have tremors or jitteriness. Seizures can take various forms as listed below. It should be noted that almost any bizarre episodic alterations of the state of the neonate may represent a seizure. The usual difficulty is in distinguishing seizure activity manifested by generalized symmetrical tonic-clonic movements from the classic tremulous movements or jitteriness. A few distinguishing clinical features can be helpful. Generalized symmetrical tonic-clonic movements are a relatively uncommon manifestation of neonatal seizures. The rhythmic movements of jitteriness or tremors are characteristically of equal amplitude and do not have a fast and slow component, as do the tonic-clonic movements of seizures. In a susceptible neonate, jitteriness or tremors are characteristically stimulus sensitive, being easily provoked by external stimuli such as a Moro reflex, noise, or simple handling, whereas seizures are not. The movements of tremors or jitteriness can usually be stopped by the examiner passively fixing the affected limb.

Tremors of high frequency and low amplitude may occur with hypoglycemia, hypocalcemia, or in an otherwise normal infant and disappear within the first week of life. Low-frequency, high-amplitude tremors are often seen in infants who have excessive activity and/or a low-threshold Moro reflex but who are otherwise normal. Coarse tremors occur as a sign of drug withdrawal in infants of addicted mothers.

The movements provoked by seizures are the most frequent and distinct neurological signs in the neonatal period. Seizure phenomena in the newborn differ greatly from those observed in older infants and children in that only rarely will newborns have well-organized symmetrical generalized tonic-clonic seizures. These differences relate to the developmental status of the neuroanatomical and physiological organization of the neonatal brain to which previous reference was made. The various neonatal seizure manifestation include:

A. Abnormal movements or alterations of tone in trunk and extremities
    1. Fragmentary clonic—multifocal, migratory (non-Jacksonian)
    2. Alternating hemiclonic
    3. Tonic
       a. Single extremity
       b. Extension of arms and legs (decerebrate)
       c. Extension of legs, flexion of arms (decorticate)
    4. Myoclonic—isolated or generalized
    5. Bicycling movements of legs
    6. Rowing or drum-beating movements of arms
    7. Loss of tone with generalized flaccidity
    8. Generalized tonic-clonic

B. Facial, oral, lingual movements
    1. Sucking
    2. Grimacing, twitching
    3. Chewing, swallowing, yawning
C. Ocular movements
    1. Tonic horizontal eye deviation
    2. Staring, blinking
    3. Nystagmoid jerks
D. Respiratory manifestations
    1. Apnea, usually preceded or accompanied by one of the other subtle manifestations of seizures
    2. Hyperapneic or stertorous breathing.

In addition to these very specific clinical manifestations, any alteration in the state of the infant which is bizarre and episodic in occurrence may be a seizure. Such activity, as mentioned previously, must be differentiated from tremor or jitteriness as well as from decerebrate or decorticate posturing. This distinction can be difficult even for the experienced clinician.

Reflexes The reflexes found to be the most useful in an initial neurological assessment include the Moro reflex, the tonic neck reflex, the placing and stepping response, sucking, the classic deep tendon reflexes, and palmar or plantar grasp. A multitude of other neonatal reflexes have been described that, although interesting, have limited value in the clinical evaluation of the neonatal nervous system. Reflexes are primarily useful when there is a consistent asymmetry identified in association with abnormal findings gained from evaluation of tone, strength, posture and movement. A reflex also can be useful in indicating CNS dysfunction if it is either obligatory or does not habituate. When either of these two conditions occurs, or when there is an absence of the commonly tested neonatal reflexes, CNS dysfunction is present.

Sensory System

The most useful sensation tested is the neonate's response to superficial pain. To optimally evaluate this sensory modality, the examiner must have the infant in a relatively quiet and preferably alert state. Testing of sensation is most important when one suspects a spinal cord, nerve root, plexus, or peripheral nerve lesion or wants to delineate the sensory level in an infant with a meningomyelocele. The nerve conduction time in both peripheral nerves and spinal cord is greatly delayed in the newborn; with a pin, there may be a delay of as long as two to three seconds before the infant responds, if he perceives the stimulus. Withdrawal of the extremitiy is a local reflex phenomenon and does not alone necessarily imply that the sensory stimulus has reached cortical awareness. Perception of sensory stimuli by the infant should include in addition to movement: crying, grimacing, alteration in respiratory pattern, change in level of consciousness, or possibly change in color. The truncal incurvation reflex (GALANT) has little value as generally applied; however, it is segmentally innervated, and local stimulation of one area of the trunk may produce local trunk incurvation, indicating that the segmental arc is intact. Therefore this reflex may be helpful in localizing a spinal cord injury.

Cranial Nerves

All the cranial nerves of a neonate can be examined easily by modifying the common neurological examination and/or by making deductions from neonatal responses involving cranial nerves.

Cranial nerve The olfactory nerve can be examined in the neonate but requires special procedures. This examination is not done during the screening examination, since its dysfunction is only rarely associated with neurological disease in the neonate.

Cranial nerve II Vision can be readily tested in the neonate, and its presence indicates that the entire visual system is intact, including the presence of a functional occipital cortex. Blinking in response to a light stimulus indicates only that the visual system is intact to the level of the superior colliculi and is not evidence of visual cortex function. Presence of vision is tested by observing the neonate fix and follow an object such as the human face through an arc of approximately 60 degrees. Since the neonate is myopic, the test object should be placed within 10 to 12 inches of the infant's face. This should be included in the neurological screening assessment of all neonates. One may elect to refine the examination of vision to determine visual acuity by producing opticokinetic nystagmus through movement of a large drum with different width black and white stripes in front of the neonate's eyes. This should usually produce some following movements of the eyes and occasionally nystagmus back in the opposite direction. With gradations of distance and width of the stripes on the drum, visual acuity can be estimated. The remaining part of the evaluation of cranial nerve II involves a thorough evaluation of the external characteristics of the eye and a funduscopic examination. The external eye findings that may be associated with diseases of the nervous system include cataracts, cloudy cornea, irregular shape or asymmetrical size of the pupil, vascular hemangioma of the sclera, and microphthalmos. Funduscopic examination is difficult but is extremely rewarding, since this is the only chance for the examiner to see actual nerve cells. The ophthalmoscope should be set at -2 to -4 diopters for the best visualization of the optic fundus. Optic disc pallor may be a normal feature, so-called pseudooptic atrophy of the newborn. Retinal hemorrhages, reported to occur in 8% to 50% of neonates, are not usually associated with significant neurological abnormalities; however, subhyaloid hemorrhages are usually associated with subdural hematomas in the infant. Retinal lesions of chorioretinitis secondary to toxoplasmosis, cytomegalovirus, rubella, or syphilis are only rarely seen in the neonatal period.

Cranial nerves III, IV, and VI The third cranial nerve must be intact for normal pupil function. The pupils should be equal and respond to light even at 28 to 30 weeks of gestation. The optimum functioning of cranial nerves III, IV, and VI connected via the medial longitudinal fasciculus can be assessed by watching the con-jugate eye movements while an infant is fixating and following. In addition, conjugate eye movements can be evaluated during the observation of normal doll's eye movement, assessed by holding the infant at arm's length in an upright posture and rotating him. This rotation stimulates the semicircular canals, and the impulses travel through the vestibular portion of cranial nerve VIII to the brainstem via the medial longitudinal fasciculus and innervate cranial nerves III and VI. This stimulation causes the eye to tonically deviate away from the direction of the rotation. Rotation should be performed in both directions. When it is impossible to rotate the neonate as mentioned, the semicircular canals may be stimulated by injecting cold water into the ear canal. In this maneuver the eyes deviate to the side of cold water injection. When the eyes remain in a fixed position regardless of stimulation or head movement, serious brainstem dysfunction is usually present. A loss of doll's eye move-ment can be seen when an excessive amount of barbiturates has been administered. A repetitive failure of the eye to move in a single direction should be noted and considered abnormal. Dysconjugate eye movements with some nystagmoid movements may not be uncommon during these maneuvers when they are performed during the first three weeks of life. However, when there is a repetitive failure of movement of the eyes in a single direction, persistent dysconjugate eye movements, or continuous nystagmus at rest, significant neurological dysfunction is present.

Cranial nerves V, VII, IX, X, XI, and XII The sensory portion of the fifth cranial nerve can be tested by eliciting the corneal reflex or using a pinprick on the face and watching for grimacing movements. In some observer's experience, the corneal reflex is not a reliable test of sensation in the newborn. The motor function of cranial nerve V is judged to be intact if the infant can close the mouth through effective masseter strength. The other cranial nerves that must be intact for an effective suck to occur are cranial nerve VII for pursing of the lips and cranial nerve XII for the milking action of the tongue. The observation of effective swallowing indicates adequate function of cranial nerves IX and X. The function of cranial nerve XI can be estimated by visualization of the sternocleidomastoid muscle when the infant is held in the supine position. There should be an ability to maintain the head in an extended position for brief periods of time. Presence of any mass in the sternocleidomastoid muscle, such as a hematoma, can be observed at this time.

Cranial nerve VIII Examination of the vestibular portion of cranial nerve VIII has been mentioned under the sections on cranial nerves III, IV, and VI. Examination of the auditory portion of this nerve can be tested in the newborn only in a gross fashion. Auditory-evoked potential using electroencephalography can now be used for more accurate testing. At the bedside, evidence of the infant's hearing can be assessed by using a graded noise stimulus. This can be either in the form of an electrical noisemaker giving a graded noise or simply a small hand bell. In confirming whether the infant hears the noise, observations either of the infant being alerted from sleep or being quieted if awake can be taken as evidence that the neonate hears. Repeated examinations may be necessary, since there may be a lack of response or a variable response of the neonate to the noise stimulus.

The importance of screening for hearing loss in early infancy is gaining wide recognition. Infants with the following conditions should be considered at risk for hearing loss:

1. Family history of childhood hearing impairment
2. Congenital perinatal infection (for example, cytomegalo-virus, rubella, herpes, toxoplasmosis, syphilis)
3. Anatomic malformations involving the head or neck (for example, dysmorphic appearance including syn-dromal and nonsyndromal abnormalities, overt or sub-mucous cleft palate, and morphological abnormalities of the pinna)
4. Birth weight less than 1500 gm
5. Hyperbilirubinemia at a level exceeding indications for exchange transfusion
6. Bacterial meningitis, especially that caused by *Hemophilus influenzae*
7. Severe asphyxia, which may be exhibited by neonates who have Apgar scores of 0-3 or who fail to institute spon-taneous respiration by 10 minutes of age, as well as by those with hypotonia persisting for two hours of age.

The screening method of choice should be dictated by the individual facility, available personnel, and number of infants to be served. However, any protocol for hearing screening to be effective must be implemented in a systematic fashion as part of an overall longitudinal follow-up program involving all infants at risk.

Interpretation of the Neurologic Assessment

The neurological assessment is particularly valuable when used to detect treatable diseases, to diagnose specific neurological disorders, and to assess gestational age. The use of the neurological assessment for the prognostic identification of neonates at risk for later abnormal development must be interpreted with caution. Except in situations where multiple unequivocal signs indicate severe damage, considerable discretion should be used in making prognostic statements. The capacity of the developing nervous system for re-organization of connections following certain kinds of injury may account for some of our inability to accurately prognosticate from abnormal neurological signs found in the neonatal period.

Even though definitive interpretation of neonatal signs of neurological dysfunction should be made with caution, the current state-of-the-art permits the following statements:

1. The full-term neonate with a negative family history, a negative prenatal, intrapartum, and neonatal history, and a normal neurological and pediatric examination has a negligible chance of subsequent abnormal neurological development related to perinatal causes.

2. Certain neurological signs, even though infrequent in their occurrence, have considerable predictive power for later abnormal neurological function. They include persistent abnormalities in tone, especially hypotonia; diminished level of activity; weak cry for more than 24 hours; and an inability to suck, requiring gavage feedings. Each of these signs carries a tenfold to twentyfold increased risk of the subsequent development of cerebral palsy. A neonate with an Apgar score of 3 or less at 10 minutes and/or neonatal seizures, especially if associated with intrapartum asphyxia and/or trauma, has a greater than fiftyfold increased risk for subsequent development of cerebral palsy.

3. Combinations of abnormalities are more significant than a single abnormality.

4. A neonate with signs of neurological dysfunction at time of discharge has a fiftyfold increased risk of having subsequent abnormal neurological development.

5. More signs of neurological dysfunction occur in a neonate who has acute damage to a previously normal nervous system than a neonate with long-standing absence of a part of the nervous system.

6. The total duration of the presence of an abnormal neurological sign does not necessarily add to or detract from its significance. Clear-cut signs of neurological dysfunction may be present for only a few days and then disappear, with the child later developing signs of frank neurological dysfunction as development progresses.

7. Asymmetrical findings are usually more significant than symmetrical findings, not so much in helping to localize the area of brain involved but simply in indicating that an underlying abnormality exists.

8. Signs of neurological dysfunction, occurring in the presence of identifiable neuropathological lesions, are more predictive of subsequent neurological abnormality than signs with no association to a demonstrable brain lesion.

There is a need for further development of more sophisticated, noninvasive techniques for identifying pathological changes in the neonatal brain, thus facilitating more accurate neonatal clinico-neuropathologic correlation and enhanced predictability of long-term sequelae from the findings of the neonatal neurological examination.

At discharge, an updated complete neurological assessment should be done, including any specific laboratory or roentgeno-graphic data relative to the nervous system. At that time the neonate should be placed in one of three categories (low-risk, high-risk, or suspect) regarding risk for subsequent delayed or abnormal development. This designation is for the purpose of planning for the child's optimum health supervision, specifically for detection of developmental delays. As stimulation programs are evaluated and deemed useful, the entry of a child into one of these programs is best done when the child first shows delay.

In using the findings from the neonatal neurological examination in counseling parents regarding the risks of subsequent abnormal neurological development, caution must be used. The physician must be honest but gentle with the parents at the time of discharge of their neonate since the child has only one set of parents.

In closing, it is important to recognize five points. The ultimate functional state of the child cannot usually be predicted accurately from the neonatal discharge examination. Most children with significant neurological dysfunction usually are cared for at home during the first seven years of life. Overt neurological dysfunction of the motor system will appear during the child's first three years of life, if the brain has sustained significant damage during the perinatal period. It may take a longer period of time, up to eight years of age, to detect abnormalities in abstract reasoning. With optimum child health supervision this child can be helped to maximize his or her assets and minimize his or her deficits.

BIBLIOGRAPHY

1. Ahmann, P. A., et al. Intraventricular hemorrhage in the high risk preterm infant: incidence and outcome. *Ann. Neurol.* 7:118, 1980.
2. American Speech and Hearing Association, American Academy of Ophthalmology and Otolaryngology, and American Academy of Pediatrics: Supplementary statement of Joint Committee on Infant Hearing Screening, *A.S.H.A. 16*:160, 1974.

3. Clark, D. B. Abnormal neurologic signs in the neonate: physical diagnosis of the newly born, In: *Report of the Forty-Sixth Ross Conference on Pediatric Research*, edited by J. Kay. 1964.
4. Dubowitz, L. M. S., Dubowitz, V., and Goldberg, C. Clinical assessment of gestational age in the newborn. *J. Pediart. 77*:1, 1970.
5. Dykes, F. D., et al. Intraventricular hemorrhage: a prospective evaluation of etiopathogenesis. *Pediatrics 66*:42, 1980.
6. Finer, N. N., et al. Hypoxic-ischemic encephalopathy in term neonates: perinatal factors and outcome. *J. Pediatr. 98*:112, 1981.
7. Goldstein, G. W. Pathogenesis of brain edema and hemorrhage: role of the brain capillary. *Pediatrics 64*:357, 1979.
8. Hagberg, B. Epidemiological and preventive aspects of cerebral palsy and severe mental retardation in Sweden. *Euro. J. Ped. 130*:71, 1979.
9. Hogan, G. R., and Ryan, N. J. Neurological evaluation of the newborn. *Clin. Perinatol. 4*:31, 1977.
10. Illingworth, R. S. *The Development of the Infant and Young Child: Normal and Abnormal*, ed. 4. Baltimore: The William and Wilkins Co., 1970.
11. Koops, B. L., and Harmon, R. J. Studies on long-term outcome in newborns with weights under 1500 grams. *Adv. Behav. Ped. 1*:1, 1980.
12. Lazzara, A., et al. Clinical predictability of intraventricular hemorrhage in preterm infants. *Pediatrics 65*:287, 1972.
13. McFarland, W. H., Simmons, F. B., and Jones, F. R. An automated hearing screening technique for newborns. *J. Speech Hearing Disorders 45*:495, 1980.
14. National Center for Health Statistics. Advance report: Final mortality statistics, 1977. *Monthly Vital Statistics Report, (Suppl.) 28(1)*, 1977.
15. Nelson, K. B., and Ellenberg, J. H. Neonatal signs as predictors of cerebral palsy. *Pediatrics 64*:225, 1979.
16. Norman, R. M. Late neuropathological sequelae of birth injury. In: *Greenfield's Neuropathology*. London: Edward Arnold Publishers, Ltd., 1964.
17. Parmalee, A. H., et al. Neurological evaluation of the premature infant. *Biol. Neonate 15*:65, 1970.
18. Prechtl, H. Prognostic values of neurological signs. *Proc. R. Soc. Med. 58*: 3, 1965.
19. Prechtl, H., and Bientema, D. The neurological examination of the full-term newborn infant. In: *Clinics in Developmental Medicine, No. 12*. London: William Heinemann Ltd., 1964.
20. Sarnat, H. B., and Sarnat, M. S. Neonatal encephalopathy following fetal distress: a clinical and electroencephalographic study. *Arch. Neurol. 33*: 696, 1976.
21. Thorne, I. Cerebral symptoms in the newborn. *Acta Paediatr. Scand. (Suppl.) 9*:15, 1975.
22. *Vital Statistics of the United States, Vol. 2, Mortality Part A*, Washington, D.C.: U.S. Government Printing Office, 1974.
23. Volpe, J. J. Neonatal seizures. *Clin. Perinatol. 4*:43, 1977.
24. World Health Organization. *Report on Social and Biological Effects on Perinatal Mortality, Vol. 1*, Geneva: WHO, 1978.

CHAPTER 10

Follow-up of the Infant Given Neonatal Intensive Care

Elsa J. Sell, M.D.

The following quotation describes a potent driving force for those interested in follow-up studies of infants who are in neonatal intensive care units (ICU):

"Our society's commitment to the saving of all ill neonates' lives entails a responsibility to maximize quality of life on the survivors." [1]

Let us consider *who should be responsible*. I would suggest at least the following: (1) parents; (2) primary health care provider, be that a pediatrician, family practitioner, public health nurse, or clinic; (3) neonatologists; (4) organized follow-up programs.

Parents should be educated about what their infant's future may bring as best we know it at the time. Otherwise, few parents would think to ask their health care provider appropriate questions at the right time. Also, it has been my experience that parents who have been educated about the possibility of a future problem cope better with the reality after a diagnosis is made. Furthermore, they will be more receptive to suggested interventions for a diagnosed problem. I cannot emphasize strongly enough that intervention will occur only if those who need it recognize and accept that need. Since our infants and young children cannot speak for themselves, they can be helped only if their parents are willing.

Perinatal Neurology and Neurosurgery. Edited by R. A. Thompson, J. R. Green, and S. D. Johnsen. Copyright © 1985 by Spectrum Publications, Inc.

Health care providers are the vital link in the chain of total care because they are the most likely to be cognizant of family, social, and environmental issues that influence childhood development. In addition, they may be the only resource following an infant who was in the ICU. Then they have a responsibility to know what to expect and how to assess the following areas: growth, neurological exam including hearing and vision, behavior, development and educational abilities.

Neonatologists' interest in a follow-up program need not be equated with management of a clinic, as few are trained for or interested in that task. However, they can assist with location of funding resources for start up and maintenance of a program. They can also encourage parent participation and be supportive of the clinic staff and program. Neonatologists should be involved with study of data from the follow-up program to learn if changes in therapy for any given problem or if new therapies alter outcome. Those fortunate neonatologists who are directly involved in follow-up programs will gain perspective of families' coping abilities, anxieties, joys, and frustrations that will be immensely helpful in supporting parents and teaching house staff and parents in the ICU. That perspective is not easily gained by reading published reports about outcome.

Finally, well organized follow-up programs can provide their communities with an expertise acquired through experience available to few individual clinics or physicians since each has a limited number of these infants in their practice. This expertise is best documented by regular data analysis and presented formally (publication in peer-reviewed journals) or informally (talks, newsletters, quarterly or yearly grant reports, or other form for the local community). I comment on this because data management should be more emphasized when planning a clinic, and it usually is not a high priority for agencies that fund primarily service-oriented follow-up programs.

How long should follow-up be? Many factors will determine this. Among the relatively uncontrollable factors are availability of funding resources and the family mobility that removes a child from the geographic region. During the organizational phase of a new follow-up program it is advisable to secure long-term commitments for funding. Controllable factors governing the length of a child's participation in the program include the end-point that one wishes to document or the service to be provided. For example, if the program were only studying neonatal behavior, the infant would be followed until the behavioral studies were completed. If the emphasis were on documentation of spastic diplegia or hemiplegia, then 9 to 12 months post-term often may be sufficiently long. If advocacy for the child and family were the primary focus, then follow until the child is functioning well in the third or fourth grade. Reference will be made to this again later.

Who should be followed? Some programs have successfully conducted epidemiological studies of complete ICU nursery populations; from these we learn about the incidence of various outcome problems. I think epidemiological studies are the most desirable for that reason. However, they are very expensive and difficult to achieve because of subject non-availability if the parents move or are no longer interested in coming to clinic. More commonly, follow-up programs have carried out epidemiological evaluation of a subset of the ICU population such as those who had respiratory distress syndrome (RDS), very low birthweight (VLBW), small-for-gestational-age (SGA) infants of diabetic mothers (IDM), birth asphyxia, intracranial hemorrhage (CH), or bronchopulmonary dysplasia (BPD).

A group that is frequently not enrolled in follow-up programs is the group who were prematurely born without significant neonatal medical problems or born at term with minimal medical problems. The low-frequency of outcome problems in these two groups seems to justify the practice. If you are the primary health care provider for such an infant, you need to be familiar with potential outcome problems and request consultation from a reliable community resource if a problem is suspected. Tables 1 and 2 illustrate two cases of larger premature infants with outcome problems.

In Table 1, the infant was referred to us at 4.5 months (adjusted age for prematurity was 3.5 months). Normally, we would have enrolled him because of ventilatory support, but did not because we were not sure of clinic funding later that year. His pediatrician

Table 1.

Birth:

35 weeks of gestation; 2700 gm; 25-year-old mother G_4 P_3; prior premature infants with RDS; assisted ventillation for 6 days; transient lethargy on day 4 home at 19 days

Development:

4½ mo — Little eye contact, delay personal-social and language development; intense thumb sucking

6 mo — Hypotonia; startles and tremors; bilateral strabismus, farsightedness; thumb sucking

Table 2.

Birth:	35 weeks of gestation; 1900 gm; 36-year-old mother G_3 P_0 SAB_2; hospitalized 3 weeks
Referral:	5 years of age
Findings:	Serous otitis media; poor fine and gross motor coordination
Outcome:	Astigmatism diagnosed and coordination improved after glasses

requested consultation. The infant had little eye contact with mother or the examiner, which is very unusual. He was delayed in personal-social and language development which also is unusual; our smallest premature infants are frequently at their chronological age in personal-social and language development on the DDST by 4 to 6 months. Intense thumb sucking is an uncommon finding which is not understood. If we can transpose experience from the neonatal period, where non-nutritive sucking seems to provide an organizational support to free the infant up for other activity, then theoretically this infant's intense sucking was a cue that his environment (the clinic, the people around him, and what we were doing with him) was extremely stressful and that he was unavailable to do more than suck. On the second visit at six months he was more hypotonic, and had bilateral strabismus, tremors, and startles that had not been noted before. He continued to display little visual interest in his surroundings, including his mother. At the time of this writing, the diagnosis was unknown.

In Table 2, preschool teacher and mother were concerned about this girl's poor motor coordination and located our clinic through friends. Her development was normal, but motor coordination was poor. Her mother called one week after the child began wearing glasses to report dramatic improvement in coordination. Adequate visual screening had not been accomplished earlier, as she lives in a rural community without a pediatrician and had not seen any health care provider because there was no acute illness. We are noticing that three- to five-year-old children are seen infrequently by health care providers. We don't know if this is an economic phenomenon or failure to schedule visits.

Next let us consider several problems within ICU units that influence interpretation of outcome results. Practices of neonatal care change with time as improved technological advances occur in the management of pregnancy, labor, delivery, and neonatal care. This has given improved survival, documented by many authors, and thus different composition of follow-up populations. In turn, outcome of infants born in the 1980s may be dissimilar to that of infants born in the 1970s.

There also is variance of management for a specific problem (for example, polycythemia and hyperviscosity) among centers within any given year. Some of these decisions may alter the mortality statistics too. For example, consider a three-day-old 700 gm infant on moderate ventilatory support who has a code arrest with the cause not identifiable (that is, is properly intubated, does not have a pulmonary air leak, and has no metabolic derrangements other than those relative to the code). What do you do now that the baby has survived five rounds of "code" medications, has a heart rate of 60 for two hours after the code, and seems comatose? All centers would have held a discussion with the parents. Some might discontinue ventilator support; others might not discontinue ventilator support unless the infant dies while on the ventilator. If the latter course were chosen and the infant survived to go home and later participate in follow-up programs, outcome data would be available; were there to be significant handicap, the prevalence of handicapping conditions for his group would be higher. If the infant died, his ICU unit would show higher mortality.

Another difficulty in comparing results from different centers is that their definitions for various problems seen in follow-up programs are not uniform. There can be deficits in growth (any or all parameters of weight, height, or head circumference), neurologically, in vision or hearing (which some would also classify as neurological problems), behaviorally, or developmentally.

Classification of outcome problems has varied among published reports. Some have placed mild or severe cerebral palsy, hydrocephalus, mental retardation, cranial nerve palsy, nystagmus, and blindness into the category of major problems and, diagnoses as minimal brain dysfunction, abnormal movements, asymmetry, detectable non-disabling tone, and reflex abnormalities as minor problems. Other investigators have more categories for handicaps (for example, profound, severe, significant, minor, none) and have utilized one or more of the following areas to determine which category: developmental scores, neurological and sensory handicaps, and

special school placement. My preference would be for such a functional classification despite the child's future dependency or indepen-
dency. We need to encourage everyone who is reporting outcome to
do so in a similar way; then we can compare results from different
centers more easily.

Some are concerned whether examiners in a follow-up program
are "blind" to the infant's/child's neonatal problems, including prematurity. It is possible to have examiners blinded to some perinatal
conditions if they do not read the medical history before performing
an evaluation. However, that will apply only to the first evaluation
for several reasons: (1) any observant examiner will remember the
child/parent pair next time; (2) any thorough service-oriented follow-
up program should have regular reviews with all staff members (we
also include our secretary). Our review includes the perinatal history,
neonatal behavioral or neurological examination, if done, prior clinic
assessments, and results of any consultations. In addition, an
examiner who has had sufficient experience (the number of children
will depend on the observational skills of the individual) will know
without looking at a medical record that an infant was a VLBW
premature infant or not. Thus, I think it is difficult to maintain
"blind" examiner status in a service oriented program, although
those that are primarily research oriented may be very successful at
achieving such status.

Next I would like to review selected studies on outcome because
of multicenter reports or the impact that perinatal factor has on a
child's future.

VERY LOW BIRTHWEIGHT

Although we are all aware of the improved mortality reported for
this group, there is uncertainty as to whether there is improved
morbidity. Stewart collated data from multiple centers between
1946 and 1977 [2]. She demonstrated improved mortality and morbidity for two groups of infants: those with birthweight below
1000 gm and those with birthweight below 1500 gm. Whether this
encouraging finding persists is questionable as some follow-up programs reflect the clinical impression that there are more handicapped
infants surviving now.

Kitchen recently published data documenting higher rates of
cerebral palsy and lower rates of visual problems in younger children
born between 1977 and 1978 versus children born from 1966 to
1970 (Table 3).

Table 3.   Comparisons of Sensorineural Handicaps in VLBW Infants from 1966–1978

	1966-1970	1977-1978
All visual deficits	32.7%	17.5%[a]
Strabismus	21.6%	12.4%
Blindness	3.9%	1.2%
Sensorineural deafness with hearing aid	3.9%	1.2%
Cerebral palsy		
mild	1.3%	5.0%
severe	2.6%	11.9%*

From Kitchen, W. H., Ryan, M. M., Rickards, A., et al. Changing outcome over 13 years of very low birthweight infants. *Seminars in Perinatology* 6:365–372, 1982.
[a]p <.05

It is unclear why the incidence of cerebral palsy was so low in the earlier period; perhaps those surviving now with cerebral palsy did not live in the earlier period. In spite of the increased neurological problems, these children had evidence of developmental catch up between two and six years (Bayley MDI and WPPSI, respectively, in Table 4).

There are an increasing number of studies on the very, very low birthweight (VVLBW) infant below 1250 or 1000 gm. I have summarized the results in Table 5. The first line shows the number seen out of the total number of survivors. The age of follow-up was chronological in all except one. Since there was variation in each paper's definition of problems, it was necessary to extrapolate a few data points so that results could be compared among centers. Survival

Table 4.   Comparison of Psychological Test Results in VLBW Infants

	1966-1970	1973-1974	1977-1978
Bayley MDI (N=64, 150)	75	—	91 (p <.05)
WPPSI (N=102, 64)	97	102	– NS

From Kitchen, W. H., Ryan, M. M., Rickards, A., et al. Changing outcome over 13 years of very low birthweight infants. *Seminars in Perinatology* 6:363–372, 1982.

Elsa J. Sell

Table 5. Outcome Problems of VVLBW Survivors

	Ruiz [4] (<1000gm)	Driscoll [5] (<1001gm)	Britton [6] (<801gm)	Hirata [7] (<750gm)	Cohen [8] (750-1000gm)	Clifford [9] (<800gm)
Number	38/40	23/26	37/39	17/22	60/75	16/19
Year of birth	1976-1978	1977-1978	1974-1977	1975-1979	1961-1980	1977-1980
Age of follow-up (mo)	8-15	8-36	15-24 posterm	24-60	36 or >	6-36
No problem in any category	53%	57%	51%	77%	67%	44%
Developmental delay, MDI 68-84	21%	19%[a]	27%	24%	17%[c]	37.5% (3/8)
Developmental delay, MDI below 68	16%	17%	22%		12%[c]	6%
Neurologic problem	21%	17%	14%	12%		6%
Vision, mild impairment	5%	17%	41%	0	?	25%
Blind or severe visual impairment	5%	4%	8%	0	3%	0
Bronchopulmonary dysplasia	37% (14/38)	35% (8/26)	14%[b] (5/37)	46% (10/22)	?	?

[a] 3/16 neurologically normal had Bayley MDI <85; 4 neurologically abnormal children were not testable.
[b] These 5 were said to have Wilson-MiKity syndrome.
[c] In this study, handicap was usually a combination of both developmental delay and neurologic problem; N=49 for developmental assessment.

Table 6. Outcome Status, VVLBW Infants, Tucson

Status	500–750gm (N=9)	751–1000gm (N=47)
Normal	2	25[a]
Mild handicap		
Development < 1SD	1[b]	3[b]
Suspect neurological		2
Suspect neurological and pulmonary problem		1
Suspect neurological and development < 1SD		4
		10
Moderate handicap		
Retinopathy of prematurity (ROP), severe		1
ROP and development < 1SD	1	3
Abnormal neurological		2
Abnormal neurological and strabismus		1
Abnormal neurological and development < 1SD		1
		8
Severe handicap		
Abnormal neurological and development < 2SD	1	1
Abnormal neurological, development < 2SD, and retinopathy of prematurity		
Unilateral ROP		1
Bilateral ROP	4	1
Congenital herpes infection		1
	5	4

[a] Includes 1 with unilateral severe RLF
[b] Includes 1 with severe strabismus

rates for those who weighed below 700 gm (not shown) ranged from zero [5] to 17% [6] and to from 58 to 63% [7]. Several authors have emphasized that VLBW infants not requiring ventilation were more likely to have a normal outcome including Cohen [8], whose three infants, below 700 gm and not ventilated, were normal. Another common observation has been that most children classified as having moderate to severe handicaps also have a concomitant neurological problem.

Unpublished results from our southern Arizona program are shown in Table 6. The period of birth was from 1976 through 1981, and the children were seen for at least 12 months (except one case who was normal at eight months) to two years. The rate of follow-up was 88%. Data beyond two years is not shown because of insufficient subject number. Only two out of nine below 751 gm were normal; unfortunately, one of those has developmental problems at age four years. Our results indicate much worse prognosis than do others' data and we don't yet know why. Outcome was much better for our infants in the 751 to 1000 gm group; 25/47 were normal and these results are similar to several studies described in the previous table. In summary, many of these studies indicate optimism, others pessimism (particularly for the tiniest ones) about outcome of the smallest survivors in our ICU nurseries.

BRONCHOPULMONARY DYSPLASIA (BPD)

Multiple perinatal factors are thought to contribute to the severity of BPD [10], a complication occurring after ventilatory assistance for newborn respiratory illness. Most important among the predisposing factors are thought to be the length of exposure to high inspired oxygen concentrations and pressure delivered by the ventilator support systems; probably an inseparable factor is the severity of lung disease requiring mechanical ventilation. The more severe the lung disease, the higher will be the ventilatory require-ments. The degree of prematurity also seems important; even the tiniest infants without RDS but requiring assisted ventilaton often have quite significant BPD. Among other factors thought to con-tribute to development of BPD are hereditary predisposition, patent ductus arteriosus with congestive heart failure, infection, intubation, ischemia, and interstitial emphysema.

BPD and extremely low birthweight are the most frequent reasons for prolonged hospitalization in the neonatal period (first 28 days of

Table 7. Description of VLBW Infants, Behavioral Study

Population (N=243)	<1500 gm and <38 weeks of gestation
Perinatal variables	BPD, RDS, CNS hemorrhage, SGA, transport
Statistical method	2 x 2 ANOVA (BPD, CHSH, RDS, SGA)
	2 x 3 ANOVA (Transport)

life) and beyond. Our program has long been interested in the behavioral characteristics of infants who have BPD because of caretaker observations of "crankiness" and other nonoptimal behavioral features. Data presented in Tables 7 and 8 were gathered in our longitudinal follow-up program from 1976 to 1981. We utilized the Brazelton Neonatal Behavioral Assessment Scale (BNBAS) modified by Als et al [11] for use in premature and other high-risk infants.

The birthweight and gestational age data are given for the comparisons between those with and without BPD and between those with and without RDS, as these two factors most frequently affect behavioral characteristics.

Tables 9 through 13 show the effect of perinatal variables on scores for the individual Brazelton items arranged in *a priori* clusters. The item score is not given, just the negative influence of the perinatal factor(s) listed. The factor that most often contributed to a lower score was BPD.

Most noticeable was that infants who had BPD were less socially capable. BPD and RDS shared influence over state control but on different items. The only effect of ICH was influence over ability to self-quiet. Parameters of physiological control were effected by both BPD and RDS. The overall summary items indicate that infants with BPD were much less vigorous, organized, or pleasant to be with.

Table 8. Neonatal Parameters

	Birthweight (gm)	Birth gestation (wk)	Gestation at test (wk)
BPD	1031[a]	28.7[a]	37.1[a]
No BPD	1259	31.0	34.1
RDS	1122[a]	29.3[a]	35.3
No RDS	1325	32.6	34.5

[a] $p < .05$ for comparison of BPD vs. no BPD or RDS vs. no RDS.

Table 9. Interactive/Social Capabilities

BNBAS item	BPD	p
Orientation		
Inanimate visual	—	c
Inanimate auditory	—	a
Animate visual	—	b
Animate auditory	—	b
Animate auditory and visual	—	c
Alertness	—	b
Cuddliness	—	b
Consolability	—	a

p: a <.05, b <.01, c<.001.
The minus sign indicates that the infants who had BPD had less optimal performance on the behavioral item.

Table 10. Motoric Capabilities

	BPD	CNSh	SGA
Reflexes			
Placing	$-^a$	$-^c$	
Rooting	$-^b$		
General tone	$-^c$		
Motor maturity	$-^b$		$-^b$
Hand-to-mouth ability	$-^b$		

p: a<.05, b<.01, c<.001.

Table 11. State Control

	BPD	CNS bleed	RDS
Rapidity of build-up			$-^b$
Irritability			$-^b$
State lability			$-^b$
Self-quieting	$-^a$	$-^a$	
Habituation			
Rattle	$-^a$		
Bell			$-^a$
Pin prick	$-^b$		

p: a<.05, b<.01, c<.001.

Table 12. Effect of Perinatal Factors on Neonatal Physiologic Control

	BPD	RDS
Tremulousness		—a
Startles	—b	—a
Skin color	—b	—b

p: a<.01, b<.001.

Now let us turn to later outcome of infants who had BPD, about whom little is known. Few centers had many survivors with BPD until the mid to late 1970s. Vohr has followed 59 children who were born between 1975 and 1977 [12]. They were divided into three groups by duration of oxygen therapy and radiological diagnosis. One group required oxygen more than 21 days and had a radiological diagnosis of BPD. Those with RDS also required oxygen more than 21 days but had no BPD radiologically. The "control" group received oxygen for less than 21 days. Birthweight and gestational age were similar in all three groups (Table 14). Respiratory illness occurred significantly more frequently and it was more severe at 4 and 12 months among the BPD group.

The neurodevelopmental outcome at two years is in Table 15. The contrast between groups is quite striking; only 24% of the BPD group was normal at two years, whereas 82 to 83% of the RDS or control groups was normal. Among those who had BPD, abnormal findings were diplegia, quadraplegia, or hydrocephalus. Only three were abnormal because of low developmental scores. In the RDS and control groups, those who were abnormal had spastic diplegia.

Cognitive abilities are in Table 16. There were no significant differences at one year, although only the control group was within the normal range (84 to 116). By two years, the children with BPD

Table 13. Overall Impression

	BPD
Attractiveness	—a
Endurance	—a
Robustness	—a
Self-organization	—a

p: a<.01.

Table 14.   Perinatal Status of VLBW Infants with BPD

	BPD (N=26)	RDS (N=8)	Control (N=25)
Birth weight, gm	1100	1055	1100
Gestation, wk	29	29	30
RDS	85%	100%	40%

From Vohr, B. R., Bell, E. F., and Oh, W. Infants with bronchopulmonary dysplasia. Growth pattern and neurologic and developmental outcome. *Am. J. Dis. Child 136*:443–447, 1982.

Table 15.   Neurodevelopmental Outcome at Two Years

	BPD[a] (N=21)	RDS (N=6)	Control (N=22)
Normal	24%	83%	82%
Suspect	24%	—	9%
Abnormal	52%	17%	9%

From Vohr, B. R., Bell, E. F., and Oh, W. Infants with bronchopulmonary dysplasia. Growth pattern and neurologic and developmental outcome. *Am. J. Dis. Child 136*:443–447, 1982.
[a] $p < .05$ for BPD vs. RDS and $< .005$ for BPD vs. control.

Table 16.   Cognitive Development at One and Two Years[a]

Age	BPD (N=14, 17)	RDS (N=3, 4)	Control (N=15, 15)
12 mos	80	73	89
23 mos	65[b]	90	91

From Vohr, B. R., Bell, E. F., and Oh, W. Infants with bronchopulmonary dysplasia. Growth pattern and neurologic and developmental outcome. *Am. J. Dis. Child 136*:443–447, 1982.
[a] Corrected for early gestation.
[b] $p < .005$ for BPD vs. RDS and BPD vs. control.

Table 17. Neonatal Characteristics

	RDS (N=98)		BPD (N=89)	
	Mean	SD	Mean	SD
Birthweight (gm)	1230	203	1030	234[b]
Gestational age (wk)	20.8	1.9	28.7	2.1[b]
Age respiratory failure (hr)	5.3	8.3	2.4	5.3[a]
Intubation, duration (hr)	232	254	610	371[b]
Oxygen administration (hr)				
21–40%	435	345	925	195[b]
<40%	99	161	357	372[b]
Hospitalization (d)	61	23	107	54[b]

[a] $p < .01$ (analysis of variance)
[b] $p < .001$

were significantly below the control group as well as more than 2 SD below the normal mean of 100. In summary, Vohr's data are glum. The majority of children with BPD had significant neurological disabilities that are thought to account for the impaired cognitive performance.

Preliminary results of our VLBW infants born between 1976 and 1980 are more encouraging. All infants had assisted ventilation for RDS or for apnea in a few of the tiniest infants. As expected those who had BPD were smaller and younger at birth and they had longer and more complicated hospitalizations (Table 17 and 18).

Clinic visits were scheduled at chronological age and not age-adjusted post-term. Clinic visits were not always possible at precisely the ages shown in Tables 19 to 21; the range was ±3 months. Those

Table 18. Neonatal Problems

	RDS percent	BPD percent
Retinopathy of prematurity	12.2	51.1[b]
Sepsis	1.0	10.6
Trachael culture positive	18.4	61.7[b]
Hydrocephalus	2.0	9.6[a]
Patent ductus arteriosus	22.4	51.1[b]

[a] $p < .05$ (X^2)
[b] $p < .001$ (X^2)

Table 19. Neurological Outcome

	RDS percent	BPD percent
Abnormal		
12 mo[a]	12.2	22.5
18 mo	10.8	13.6
24 mo	16.7	15.4
Normal		
12 mo	67.3[b]	50.0
18 mo	78.4	63.6
24 mo	70.8	61.5

[a]The first N is for the group with RDS, the second
N for the BPDers
    12 mo N=49, 40;
    18 mo N=37, 22;
    24 mo N=24, 13;
[b]The remaining children had suspect neurologic
exams.

Table 20. Cognitive Development, Corrected for Gestational Age

Age	RDS		BPD	
	Mean	SD	Mean	SD
12 mo (N=44 RDS; 41 BPD)	112	24	107	31
18 mo (N=40 RDS; 27 BPD)	108	18	100	27
24 mo (N=34, RDS; 18 BPD)	100	19	93	24

Table 21. Motor Development, Corrected for Gestational Age

Age	RDS		BPD	
	Mean	SD	Mean	SD
12 mo (N=44 RDS; 41 BPD)	97	21	89	26
18 mo (N=40 RDS; 27 BPD)	95	26	96	23
24 mo (N=34, RDS; 18 BPD)	95	22	95	21

two factors may explain why the percentage of abnormal neurological exams was somewhat higher at 12 months in those with BPD, although the differences were not significant.

Developmental outcome was assessed with the Bayley Scales of Infant Development, and correction was made for early gestational age of both groups.

Our results are more encouraging than Vohr's. The cognitive and motor scores were within the normal range for both the RDS and BPD groups. Note that the scores were highest in cognitive development at 12 months. We have observed this in all groups under study. Correction for early gestational age seems to overcorrect the youngest children's cognitive scores well above the norm mean. In contrast, adjustment of motor scores for early gestation just brings them closer to the mean at all three ages.

SMALL-FOR-GESTATIONAL-AGE (SGA)

The impact of this perinatal problem on outcome has been studied more than that of BPD. Among the earliest reports was Fitzhardinge's on 96 full-term infants born between 1960 and 1966 [13]. Major neurological problems were uncommon although approximately 25% had signs of cerebral dysfunction defined as one or more of the following: hyperactivity, short attention span, learning difficulties, or poor fine motor coordination. IQ was in the average range, yet 50% of male and 36% of female children demonstrated poor school performance.

Harvey recently reported that the rate of intrauterine head growth influenced later development in term infants (N=51) at a mean age of five and one tenth years (range, 3 to 7) [14]. Each SGA infant was matched with an average-for-gestational-age infant for sex, social class, birth order, and birth date within six months. Infants were excluded if they had congenital anomalies, symptomatic hypoglycemia, or congenital viral infection. The SGA study group was subdivided into those who had decrease of head growth before or after 26 weeks of gestation. There were 10 in the early growth retardation group, 23 with later growth failure, and 18 with no growth failure. The latter two groups (later and no growth failure) were combined because they showed no subgroup differences and were designated late growth failure. Both early and late failure groups were compared to their own controls and to each other (Table 22).

Table 22.   McCarthy Scores of SGA Children

Test scale	Early growth retardation (N=10)	Late growth retardation (N=41)
Perceptual performance[a]	52	58
Quantitative[a]	49	56
Motor[a]	45	51
General Cognitive Index[b]	103	113

[a]N=50 ± 10.
[b]N=100 ± 16.

From Harvey, D., Prince, J., Braton, J., et al. Abilities of children who were small-for-gestational-age babies. *Pediatrics 64*:296–300, 1982.

There were significant differences on three of five McCarthy subscales and the General Cognitive Index. Thus it appears possible to predict a child's future by performing sequential fetal ultrasound measurement of head growth beginning before 26 weeks of gestation. Separate studies showed that the earlier growth retardation group had perceptual problems and difficulty with tests of coordination and balance [15], and school teacher's assessment showed that they had more reading and writing difficulties, particularly among the boys who were also thought to be clumsy [16].

Neligan published a study of multiple possible factors that could influence outcome of prematurely and growth retarded infants [17]. Social and environmental factors, which are known to influence later childhood development, were evaluated along with perinatal factors for influence on cognitive, behavioral, neurological and growth parameters at five, six, and seven years of age. Table 23 summarizes his study. Those interested in follow-up should be acquainted with this book.

Table 23.   Neligan Study of Infant Born Too Soon or Too Small

1. Both short-gestation and those SGA performed significantly less well than controls at 5, 6, 7 years.

2. The degree of intrauterine growth impairment is proportional to the degree of impairment of later performance.

3. Overall performance of those SGA is significantly worse than the short-gestation group.

4. Impaired performance of both groups persists even when biological, clinical, and environmental factors are considered.

Tooley's group has found some differences in IQ scores of VVLBW infants according to whether or not there was intrauterine malnutrition. Those who were SGA and in the weight groups below 800 gm and between 800 to 899 gm, had lower scores than AGA babies of the same weight [18]. The SGA and AGA infants of 900 to 999 gm had similar IQ scores.

So, both term and some VVLBW preterm SGA infants have lower IQ scores. Whether our obstetrical colleagues will be able to diminish this difficulty with earlier diagnosis and new management of intrauterine fetal malnutrition, remains to be seen. At least neonatologists and primary health care providers should do their best to educate such infants' parents early on that longitudinal assessment into school age will be important.

INTRACRANIAL HEMORRHAGE (ICH)

One of the most exciting recent technological advances has been the diagnostic ability to document non-invasively that ICH has or has not occurred even in the sickest neonate. Investigators have reported their results at the two intracranial hemorrhage conferences sponsored by Ross Laboratories in Washington, D.C. I have selected data from Papile [19] as she is among the pioneers in clinical studies on ICH. I would recommend reading the conference syllabus to those of you particularly interested in ICH. All infants in Papile's study were VLBW; birthweight and gestational age (Table 24) were similar for the control group and the groups with ICH, regardless of the grade of bleeding. Outcome is given in Table 25.

The incidence of problems was similar in infants with no bleeding and those with grade I or II hemorrhage; major handicap was found in 11% and normal status in 39 to 49%. Those with grade III and IV

Table 24. Birthweight and Gestational Age of VLBW Infants with ICH

	No bleed	Grade I	Grade II	Grade III	Grade IV
Number	115	33	19	14	17
Birthweight, gm	1180	1070	1120	1140	1060
Gestational age, wk	30.2	29.2	29.4	28.9	2.1

From: Papile, L., Munsick–Bruno, G., and Schaefer, A. The relationship of cerebral intraventricular hemorrhage and early childhood neurologic handicaps. *The Second Special Ross Laboratories Conference on Perinatal Hemorrhage, Vol. III*, 1982.

Table 25. Percentage Outcomes of VLBW Infants with ICH

	No bleed	Grade I	Grade II	Grade III	Grade IV
Normal	49	42	39	29	12
Handicap					
Minor	40	46	50	14	6
Major	11	12	11	57	82

From: Papile, L., Munsick–Bruno, G., and Schaefer, A. The relationship of cerebral intra-ventricular hemorrhage and early childhood neurologic handicaps. *The Second Special Ross Laboratories Conference on Perinatal Hemorrhage, Vol. III*, 1982.

bleeding had more major handicaps that increased with severity of the bleeding. Papile has also documented more handicapping problems in infants who have hydrocephalus after ICH, with approximately 75% abnormal.

Since the overall frequency of ICH in VLBW infants is close to 50% and outcome is dependent upon the severity of bleeding and the subsequent development of hydrocephalus, it has become routine for all VLBW infants to have head ultrasound examinations at regular intervals. Presently available data suggest that ultrasound done at 4, 7, and 14 days will detect the majority of bleeding. Additional studies are indicated whenever head growth occurs more rapidly than body growth, although this should be infrequently needed if there are regularly scheduled exams. After two weeks, examinations are done to follow the progression of porencephalic cyst formation after grade IV bleeding, development of and changes in hydrocephalus, and to occasionally document new ICH. We do not yet understand why some infants with severe bleeding have normal outcome and others, abnormal outcome. Even so, neonatologists and pediatricians involved in intensive care can discuss future outcome of infants with ICH more accurately than was possible six years ago. We should realize that the final answer is not yet in with respect to later development in youngsters who had minor bleeding and seem to be normal in the first several years of life.

SCHOOL-AGE ABILITIES

Although much has been learned about early outcome of ICU nursery graduates, I think that the most pertinent end-point is the child's ability to function in school as demands become more complex with increasing grade. Now there are some tremendous hurdles to be overcome by investigators who carry their studies this far. Longitudinal studies take time and that can create academic discomfort (no publications) for those in university settings. Publication of early-onset problems is appropriate particularly if the topic is a new problem or approach. However, early publication can be misleading if there are few or no problems, implying that all is well; practitioners then become complacent and don't worry about the children as they become older. Another difficulty in conducting long-term studies is that few funding agencies understand the value of such work nor are they willing to commit funds for an extended period. Finally, individuals in a program may disappear and reappear at unplanned times because of family mobility and/or interest. This can wreak havoc with statistical analyses for which one needs data filling all time points. However, it is better to see the children for an assessment than not at all!

There are several papers in the literature on school outcome of children born in the 1950s and 1960s [20,21]. For our purposes it is best to review the most recent papers. The first from England was on VLBW infants born between 1968 and 1975 [22]. Only 33% of the survivors were seen; however, the study is important because all children were considered normal by their families and most had been classified as normal on earlier follow-up examination. There were 23 VLBW children matched for age, sex and social class with 23 term controls selected at random. The mean age of follow-up was 9.1 years for both groups. A neurological exam adpated from Touwen is given in Table 26; higher neurological scores indicate more abnormality. A neurological score above five was found in no controls but in 8/23 of the premature infants. The latter also did less well on 4/5 subtests of the revised WISC-R; verbal IQ, performance IQ, and full-scale IQ. Remember, these premature infants had been considered normal.

Hunt investigated learning disabilities in a group of VLBW children, 85% of whom were available for complete evaluation through four years of age [23]. The families were middle class and lived in the San Francisco area. The incidence of learning disabilities was 37%. There was a small control group of siblings who were not low birthweight and were evaluated at age four years or older. Sixteen sibling pairs were tested and the average IQ was 16.7 points higher in the controls. At six years, 49% of the VLBW children had disability in language comprehension or visual-motor integration skills or both. Most interesting was a comparison of six- and eight-year abilities,

Table 26. Neurological Scoring Criteria, Comparison of Two Recent Studies

	Score = 1	Score = 2
Cranial nerves		
Visual activity	<6/6 One eye	<6/7.5 Both eyes
Fundi	Increased tortuosity of arteries	Abnormal
Other	Mild	Gross
Power	One limb slightly weak	One limb very weak
		>One limb affected
Tone	—	Abnormal
Sensation	—	Abnormal
Skeletal kyphosis, scoliosis, or contractures	Slight abnormality	Definite abnormality
Reflexes	Asymmetry or recruitment	Marked asymmetry or clonus
Walking	Broad based gait	Gross abnormality
	Abduction of arms	
	Intoeing	
On toes	Few steps only	Gross abnormality
	Associated movements	
On heels	Difficulty raising toes	Unable to raise toes

Standing on one leg	Foot down <5 sec	Unable to do
Involuntary movements	Choreiform or athetoidiform mov. at 2–5/20 sec.	6–10 Movements/20 sec
Pronation of arms		
With eyes shut	Slight deviation or spooning	Marked deviation or spooning
	Slight associated movements	Marked imbalance
Push eyes shut	Moves	Falls
Hop on 1 foot	Poor balance	Cannot do
Diadochokinesis	Elbow moves > 15 cm	Grossly abnormal
Mouth opening	Slight finger spread	Marked finger spread and wrist extension
Finger–nose	Tremor or misses once	Marked tremor or miss more than once
Finger opposition	Misses finger sequence, wrong mirror movements	Frequent misses, marked associated movements

From Noble–Jamieson, C. M., Lukeman, D., Silverman, M., and Davies, P. M. Low birthweight children at school age: neurological, psychological and pulmonary function. *Seminars in Perinatology 6*:266–273, 1982.

Table 27. IQ Comparisons at 4–6 and 8 Years (N=53)

	Four-six years	Eight years		
		Normal	Suspect	Abnormal
IQ < 68	2			2
IQ 68–83	10			10
IQ > 84				
Handicap	10		3	7
Suspect	11	4	3	4
Normal	20	9	7	4

From Hunt, J. V., Tooley, W. H., and Harvin, D. Learning disabilities in children with birth weights <1500 grams. *Seminar in Perinatology 6*:280–287, 1982.

shown in Table 27. The children who had been retarded or border-line at six years continued to be so classified at eight years. Those who had normal IQs at six years had diverse future performance. About one-third with abnormal global ratings had improvement in that rating although the average IQ was not improved. About equal numbers of those considered suspect showed shifts to better or poorer status. An unexpected finding was that only four of the 20 children who had been considered normal remained normal. Their shift downward in level (for example, from normal to suspect or abnormal) was also accompanied by a decline in IQ. We should pay attention to the findings that learning disabilities continue to be identified beyond the first grade and in children who were thought to be normal earlier.

Kitchen followed 159 VLBW infants to age eight and five infants to age six years [24]. Few (N=8) attended special schools, the placement of five was not known, and the others were in normal school. Handicaps were profound in 5.1% of the infants, severe in 10.8%, significant in 40.5% of the VLBW group; a normal birthweight comparison group had 2.3% profound, 0% severe, and 25.6% with significant handicap. Among the VLBW group, 15.9% were either not reading or were retarded by more than 18 months and the full-scale WISC-R IQ was 88.8 as compared to 98.8 for the normal birth-weight group.

We too find that a high percentage (32/73 or 44%) of school-age children are having a school problem, defined as the need to repeat a grade or receiving special educational/learning assistance, or both. Furthermore, we have been able to predict 75% of the children with a school problem from the children's performance on the McCarthy scales of children's abilities at both four and five years. This is very exciting information but we have additional factors that need investigation, such as the effect of maternal educational level and whether discrepancies on certain subscales of the four- and five-year McCarthy scale (for example, perceptual performance vs. quantitative skills) are also highly predictive of school problems.

In final summary, we can say that outcome of the newborn given care in the ICU nursery is laced with both certainties and uncertainties. How do we cope with helping each child reach his fullest potential? The least we can do is educate the parents about what the future may hold. This needs to be done discreetly so as to not overly alarm the parents, yet to have them informed. It should be done with the emphasis that parental expectations and hopes for their child as well as opportunities for learning will influence the future. Ideally, we would follow each ICU infant into middle school, identifying any problems along the way. What can be accomplished in reality depends upon parental motivation and the available diagnostic and therapeutic resources of the community.

REFERENCES

1. Friedman, S., Chipman, S. F., Segal, J. W., and Cocking, R. R. Complimenting the success of medical intervention. *Seminars in Perinatology 6*: 365-372, 1982.
2. Stewart, A. L., Reynolds, E. O. R., and Lipscomb, A. P. Outcome for infants of very low birth weight; survey of world literature. *Lancet* 1038-1041, May 1981.
3. Kitchen, W. H., Ryan, M. M., Rickards, A., et al. Changing outcome over 13 years of very low birthweight infants. *Seminars in Perinatology 6*:373-389, 1982.
4. Ruiz, M. P. D., LeFever, J. A., Hakanson, D. O., et al. Early development of infants of birth weight less than 1000g with reference to mechanical ventilation in newborn period. *Pediatrics 68*:330-335, 1981.
5. Driscoll, J. M., Driscoll, Y. T., Steir, M. E. et al. Mortality and morbidity in infants less than 1001g birth weight. *Pediatrics 69*:21-26, 1982.
6. Britton, S. B., Chir, B., Fitzhardinge, P. M. et al. Is intensive care justified for infants weighing less than 801g at birth? *J. Pediatrics 99*:937-943, 1981.
7. Hirata, T.: Personal communication, 1981.
8. Cohen, R., Stevenson, D. K., Malachowski, N. et al. Favorable results of neonatal intensive care for very low birth weight infants. *Pediatrics, 69*: 621-625, 1982.
9. Bennett, F. C., Robinson, N. M., and Sells, C. J. Growth and development of infants weighing less than 800g at birth. *Pediatrics 71*:319-323, 1983.

10. Taussig, L. Bronchopulmonary dysplasia. In: *Follow-up of the High Risk Newborn—A Practical Approach*, edited by E. Sell. Springfield, Illinois: Charles C Thomas, 1980.
11. Als, H., Tronick, E., and Brazelton, T. B. *Manual for the Behavioral Assessment of the Premature and At-Risk Newborn.* Unpublished manuscript, 1976.
12. Vohr, B. R., Bell, E. F., and Oh, W. Infants with bronchopulmonary dysplasia. Growth pattern and neurologic and developmental outcome. *Am. J. Dis. Child 136*:443-447, 1982.
13. Fitzhardinge, P. M., and Steven, E. M. The small-for-date infant. II. Neurological and intellectual sequelae. *Pediatrics 50*:50-57, 1972.
14. Harvey, D., Prince, J., Bruton, J. et al. Abilities of children who were small-for-gestational-age babies. *Pediatrics 64*:296-300, 1982.
15. Wallis, S., Shamsi, D., and Harvey, D. Neurological examination of children who were small-for-dates babies: In: *Poor Intrauterine Fetal Growth*, edited by B. Salvadori and A. Bacchi Modena. Rome: Centro Minerva Medica, 1977.
16. Parkinson, C. E., Wallis, S., Harvey, D. School achievement and behavior of children who were small-for-dates at birth. *Develop. Med. Child Neurol. 23*:41-50, 1981.
17. Neligan, G. A., Kolvin, I., Mel. Scott, D., Garside, R. F. *Born Too Soon or Born Too Small.* Philadelphia: Spastics International Medical Publications, J. B. Lippincott Co., 1976.
18. Tooley, W. Medical and psychomotor development of children with birthweight less than 1000g. Presented at Annual Pediatric Update CME Course, Tucson, AZ, 1982.
19. Papile, L., Munsick-Bruno, G., and Schaefer, A. The relationship of cerebral intraventricular hemorrhage and early childhood neurologic handicaps. *The Second Special Ross Laboratories Conference on Perinatal Hemorrhage, Vol. II*, 1982.
20. Rubin, R. A., Rosenblatt, C., and Balow, B. Psychologic and educational sequelae of prematurity. *Pediatrics 52*:352-363, 1973.
21. Wiener, G. The relationship of birth weight and length of gestation to intellectual development at ages 8 to 10 years. *J. Pediatrics 76*:694-699, 1970.
22. Noble–Jamieson, C. M., Lukeman, D., Silverman, M., and Davies, P. M. Low birthweight children at school age: neurological, psychological and pulmonary function. *Seminars in Perinatology 6*:266-273, 1982.
23. Hunt, J. V., Tooley, W. H., and Harvin, D. Learning disabilities in children with birth weights <1500 grams. *Seminars in Perinatology 6*:280-287, 1982.
24. Kitchen, W. H., Ryan, M. M., Rickards, A., et al. A longitudinal study of very low birth weight infants. IV. An Overview of Performance at Eight Years of Age. *Develop. Med. Child Neurol. 22*:172-188, 1980.

CHAPTER 11

Ethical and Economic Issues

H. Belton P. Meyer, M.D.

Advances in medical sciences and technology have nearly eliminated many life-threatening diseases in the modern world and have greatly reduced the morbidity along with the mortality [1]. For a significant proportion of mankind, advances in medicine and in other phases of our lives have led to a growing expectation of health and life-style that result in increasing assumptions and sense of power over the quality of our lives. It therefore seems the more tragic to us when some of us are born with, or acquire as newborns, those conditions for which our technology has promoted survival, but with no hope for cure. In a world that appears to be so much under our control, afflicted persons confront us with the limits of our power, and, in our frustration, we may become increasingly motivated to exercise freedom of choice over the fate of those for whom we feel responsible.

As we move beyond the science and art of curing and further into the realm of caring, while controlling the instruments of life and death, the grounds for our decision-making come to be weighted heavily in the moral-ethical, in addition to the scientific, dimensions of the medical fold. But doctors and all health care professionals are much more specifically prepared in thier scientific and technical skills and are justified in their unease with exercising ethical responsibility. It is desirable that this unease will tend to lead more often to a humbler perspective and a desire to learn and share responsibility rather than provoke rash action. It is similarly desirable that the challange to devise ingenious mechanisms for care will come to match the zeal to cure.

Perinatal Neurology and Neurosurgery. Edited by R. A. Thompson, J. R. Green, and S. D. Johnsen. Copyright © 1985 by Spectrum Publications, Inc.

Moral and ethical concerns engendered by our industrialized and now high-tech society are not new. A keynote for this discussion on ethics and costs was eloquently expressed over 100 years ago by Dr. Andrew Combe in his "Treatise on the Physiological and Moral Management of Infancy" [2].

> Here then is unquestionable evidence of the fact that a great mortality prevails in infancy, even among the most civilized communites, and under what are considered the most favorable circumstances; and the question naturally presents itself, whether this mortality constitutes a necessary part of the arrangements of Divine Providence which men can do nothing to modify, or, on the contrary, proceeds chiefly from secondary causes purposely left, to a considerable extent, under our control, and which we may partially obviate or render innocuous by making ourselves acquainted with the nature of the infant constitution, and carefully adapting our conduct to the laws or conditions under which its different functions are intended to act?

> If we consult the past history of mankind, there will be little difficulty in finding the true reply, and proving that the appalling waste of infant life is not a necessary and intentional result of the Divine arrangements, but is produced chiefly by our own ignorance and mismanagement, and consequently may be expected to diminish in proportion as our knowledge and treatment improve, or, in other words, in proportion as we shall discover and fulfill the laws which the Creator has established for our guidance and preservation.

> The average mortality of infants among rich and poor is about one in every four-and-one-half before the end of the first year of existence. So directly, however, is infant life influenced by good or bad management, that, about a century ago, the workhouses of London presented the astounding result of twenty-three deaths in every twenty-four infants under the age of one year! For a long time this frightful devastation was allowed to go on as beyond the reach of human remedy. But when at last an improved system of management was adopted, in consequence of a parliamentary inquiry having taken place, the proportion of deaths was speedily reduced to 450 a year. Here then, was a total of 2150 instances of loss of life, occurring yearly in a single institution, chargeable, not against any

unalterable decrees of Providence, as some are disposed to contend as an excuse for their own negligence, but against the ignorance, indifference, or cruelty of man! And what a lesson of vigilance and inquiry ought not such occurrences to convey, when even now, with all our boasted improvements, every tenth infant still perishes within a month of its birth?

In the race of life, the chances are greatly in favor of the well-constituted and healthy, and against the badly constituted and infirm child. And yet we not infrequently see the delicate and sickly child, under good management turn out a healthy and vigorous adult; while its more promising companion has either disappeared from the scene, or become enfeebled in health, and unfit for the business of life. If a weak child can in some instances be thus strengthened, and a vigorous child lost, what stronger proof can be required that health is to a considerable extent, influenced by our own conduct and management? Surely the same good treatment which restored the feeble child should have been equally efficacious in preserving the strong, if duly adapted to its constitution?

The grand principle is that human life was not intended to be extinguished at its very dawn; this is always from the operation of previously existing causes, some of which might have been discovered and removed, while others, if not entirely counteracted, at least might have been partially subdued.

We, like Dr. Combe, must be concerned with the care of human life and, caring, to preserve all its potential. I would most like to emphasize these positive aspects of caring in this essay. But we must also address the issues of how to develop knowledge and sensitivity to *properly* use skills that are virtually unlimited toward sustaining life, but tragically limited in terms of cure of disease and enhancement of the quality of life. Multiple complex problems presented by newborns with defects or severe perinatal complications have discouraged some physicians from applying the available intensive medical care and technologies to preserve lives of the more severely defective newborns with these defects. A number of physicians have advocated strongly that treatment be withheld from newborns presenting certain criteria, with the expectation that these babies would soon die. Concerns have been expressed that the quality of life promoted by vigorous intervention might constitute a "fate worse than death," and it has been posited, "Even if all the infants saved were destined to grow up as perfectly normal human beings we would still have to face the fundamental moral question of whether the large expenditure of skilled medical and nursing time, as well as the monetary expense, is justifiable when so much needs to be done to save the lives of children all over the world" [3].

In this essay, I present some views regarding the concept of selection for treatment or non-treatment for conditions afflicting newborns with birth defects, consideration of the nature of the lives of these infants, the roles of significant actors in the decision-making process, and some reflections on the quality of life questions, including cost considerations. Additionally, I touch on some of the obligations we may properly have toward individuals with multiple handicaps who will survive and on how meeting these obligations may influence the early decisions of how far to go with initial vigorous supportive techniques.

For our time, the condition that has been most thoroughly debated in these areas that jointly concern pediatricians, child neurologists and neurosurgeons is myelodysplasia, most commonly expressed as spina bifida.

Before taking up the medical-ethical issues inherent in the approach to myelodysplasia in the newborn, I wish to offer a few observations regarding technology—its risks and benefits: It is popular in the late 20th century to enjoy the ill health of a hangover of remorse and disillusion following a binge of technological progress. We love to agonize over the unpleasant side effects and fall-out from scientific and technological applications. This, in part, represents a developmental maturation of healthy respect for the evil as well as good potential in awesome powers. But we can easily become over-burdened with dread and forget the positive benefits. So we should not forget that infant and maternal mortality have fallen progressively in this century, in part due to social change, in part attributable to medical progress. Newborn intensive care has been so much more effective in limiting cerebral palsy that the enormous improvements in survival of very low-birthweight infants appear to be associated with a greater proportionate reduction in lifelong handicaps even in very high risk groups. Most recently, non-invasive examination of intracranial anatomy and physiology has dramatically increased our knowledge of pathophysiology of cerebral hemorrhages. The result is that intraventricular hemorrhages which we formerly thought to be due only to the vulnerability of the immature to birth asphyxia and trauma, are now monitored so closely that we discover those events in the nursery that can initiate these bleeds and can avoid them. We have recently reduced the incidence of periventricular/intraventricular hemorrhage in a very low-birthweight population locally from a high of 85% to one of 20 to 25%. This is especially pertinent to our discussion today. In the past, in very low-birthweight infants on respirators with the severest Grade IV hemorrhages, we first discovered a syndrome of impending death so clearly delineated that it became relatively easy to justify discontinuing support that we could all recognize as extraordinary in interfering with the process of dying. More recently, a discouraging condition that we formerly perceived to be inevitable proved to be preventable when thoroughly investigated through applied technology. Another example is our experience with providing mechanical ventilatory support for infants of birthweights less than 1000 gm with respiratory failure. In 1970, my associate Dr. William Daily, reviewing the world literature, could find not a single instance of survival through these techniques in this birthweight category [4]. Many held that any infant survivor of this birthweight would have a high probability of severe handicaps in future life. We seriously considered withholding ventilator support from these terribly vulnerable infants, under the justification that undocumented success made such support experimental in nature. Beginning immediately thereafter, throughout the early 1970s, a progressive accumulation of literature documented a largely favorable prognosis for the survivors, and we were able to report a survival rate of nearly 50% among the ventilated babies by 1974 [5]. Now, in 1983, there is widespread experience of approximately 50% survival among those infants with birthweight between 500 and 750 gm. Nearly all of these infants must be ventilated to survive. The early follow-up to these survivors demonstrates a higher risk for significant impairment than in higher birthweight categories but may appear intact [6].

Turning to the medical-ethical problem of how to select the most appropriate treatment for the individual patient with myelodysplasia, I am indebted to Dr. David Shurtleff of the University of Washington Department of Pediatrics and Head of the Division of Congenital Defects for an outstanding treatment of the "Attitudes, Causes and Consequences" of myelodysplasia, in his excellent monograph, "Myelodysplasia: Management and Treatment in *Current Problems in Pediatrics* published in January, 1980 [7]. I commend this monograph to all concerned with this subject for its comprehensive treatment of all phases of care, based upon a vast experience and presented in a most lucid, orderly, and practical manner. I can do no better to frame the issues in myelodysplasia than to offer a synopsis of Shurtleff's review.

Historical background and multicultural attitudes in our society must be reviewed if we are to comprehend what we are about to do as we undertake care. We must be cognizant that economics do directly affect the type of treatment of children with myelodysplasia in the United States and that the cultural background of pediatricians and neurosurgeons have influenced their attitudes toward newborns with defects.

As reviewed by Bakan [8], social attitudes toward the worth of the child, whether normal or malformed, were initiated during prehistory and have been recorded in a variety of ways. Spartans were notable in their elimination of infants with defects. In the 1700s Malthus' theory predicted the inability of society to support its larger number of children, normal or abnormal. Darwin, in the 19th century stated that society was now too humane ever to regress to such barbaric concepts as abortion and infanticide:

> These practices appear to have originated in savages recognizing the difficulty, or impossibility, of supporting all infants that are born.

During the latter half of the 19th century, attitudes toward persons with defects generally followed the trends of prevention of cruelty to children coincident with the rapidly expanding industrialization of Europe and the resultant availability of goods and services.

To illustrate how recent are our social mechanisms protecting children and the shift in our concepts of the nature of the relationships of children to their parents, a brief anecdote is appropriate here.

In Boston, in the 1870s, a settlement worker, investigating a report, entered a home to discover a 13-year-old girl roped to a bedpost. There was gross evidence of physical abuse and subsequently sexual abuse was proven, all perpetrated upon her by her stepfather. The settlement worker sought relief for the girl through court action, but was frustrated by the lack of any law to intervene on behalf of the child, if action was required against the parents' prerogatives. The prevailing cultural view, supported by the law, was that children were a form of property—chattel of their parents, permitting the parents the broadest latitude in treatment of their children, short of killing them. The settlement worker succeeded in obtaining court restraint of the abuse of this girl, appealing to the existing laws preventing cruelty to animals. In association with this action, a pioneer organization toward the establishment of child protection authority was formed in Boston. It was called the Society for Prevention of Cruelty to Children, patterned after the pre-existing Society protecting animals.

In the 20th century, preoccupation with eugenics reintroduced an attitude favoring the killing of defective children. (Please note the nuance: "defective children" vs. "children with defects.") The Nuremburg Trials condemned Pfannmueller and other German physicians for their part in starving to death handicapped children [9]. There is concern that acceptance of the reintroduction of the concept of selecting children for non-treatment on the basis of their value to society as advocated by Lorber represents a turn toward the attitudes that permitted the German physician's actions [10]. Shurtleff points out that the responding *medical* arguments about selective treatment have chiefly been about the particular criteria, not about the concept [7].

The principles behind the procedure for selection for non-treatment as described by several authors are to look at large groups of patients and determine that a child is better off dead than mentally retarded with or without physical handicap to the point that the individual cannot engage in the usual social activities and will be a burden to family and society. The authors have determined that the child is "too costly" to society and advocate that the funds be better spent for more minor conditions afflicting a larger number of persons [7]. Among other criticisms of this logic, Shurtleff cites Veatch's argument in his discussion of "the technical criteria fallacy" [11]. He observes that many physicians are becoming "so infatuated with our technical abilities to accumulate data and tally scores that we run the risk of seriously misunderstanding the nature of the difficult decisions that must be made" [8]. Physicians have pointed out this ethical fallacy by describing the unpredictability of selection criteria [12-14]. We are incapable of accurately predicting in any given case either the ultimate outcome of a "good candidate" or whether a severely affected child will thrive. Death may be promoted by a passive involuntary euthanasia that is widely practiced, though of questionable legality; but it can only be assured by a process of clearly illegal active euthanasia. Many authors report 10-20% survival of children selected for non-treatment [7].

Comparison of the various medical reports regarding technical criteria reveals little agreement as to the specific criteria, or how properly to use them, given practical and theoretical difficulties. The disagreements among ethicists are no less impressive. But it can be identified that many persuasive ethical arguments converge upon a point of agreement with Shurtleff—one that I agree with; he recommends, as an alternative to a utilitarian ethic, a policy of basing decisions only on what is best for the child [7]. In this we are joined in advocacy by DeLange [15], Rickham [12], and John Freeman [16]. The considerations for treatment should be based on an understanding of the anatomy of the lesion, its physiological consequence, and what might be expected as a result of treatment.

Many of the early approaches led to serious complications of treatment. Other treatments will be to no avail: back closure will not benefit mental development in a child with associated CNS malformations; a shunt will not guarantee intellect for a child whose brain has been malformed or whose brain has cortical destruction from bleeding into the brain or infection.

Shurtleff's approach is to recognize these variables and opt for treatments for the child based on value of the treatment to the infant rather than according to "selection criteria for non-treatment" [7]. He finds this approach helpful in resolving a set of potentially conflicting interests:

- of the infant, for self-preservation and the enjoyment of life;
- of the parents, affectionate concerns and a sense of responsibility, as over and against the burdens of care of a handicapped child;
- of the state, interested in the proper fulfillment of responsibilities and duties regarding the well-being of the infant, versus the cost of provision of medical care, habilitative support, and education;
- of the treatment "team" which is concerned with the duty to take medical measures conducive to the well-being of the baby, but also with the frustration of dealing with depressing results, or responding to the temptation to enhance personal reputations.

Defining the value of the treatment to the child must balance the pain of that treatment, the degree to which it may radically interfere with the child's ability to develop relationships with its parents or consistent loving caretakers, and the ultimate benefits to the child in terms of relief of pain and suffering and improvement in health and well-being. It is easy to decide in favor of treatments that relieve pain or improve physical performance. The needs of the child must be understood and remain central when a back is closed, or a "social shunt" placed, insofar as these facilitate the opportunity for a positive relationship to natural or foster parent or nurse. The infant's interests might be poorly served if prolonged, repeated, painful hospital treatments accomplish no more than lengthening a short life span with no relief of dependency from continuous medical care and with suffering persistent separation from loving parents.

Rather than a list of criteria, Shurtleff describes a "process" of making a legal, moral, and ethical decision to treat, or to refrain from operating on, a child [7]. He dissects this process into its elements and flow. The process begins with presentation for assessment by the family and the patient with a defect. This is followed by expert and competent assessment. Assessment is followed by an informed consent conference, which leads to a decision acceptable to all in the vast majority of cases. Discussion at this level should include the physician evaluation, prognosis, and recommended plan of action. These should be clearly communicated to and discussed with the parents or guardian of the infant and with their selected close friends and advisors. Alternatives should be discussed. A sense of the parents' acceptance or rejection should be appreciated and the parents' wishes should be followed unless the physician recognizes that the parents' decision is based on their own interests at the expense of the child.

Various possibilities emerge from the informed consent conference, leading through varying paths.

In one instance physician and parents agree upon treatment, which then proceeds and is accomplished by appropriate follow-up, that is, on-going assessment and reassessment.

In a second instance physician and parents agree upon withholding some form of treatment. A program for continuing care still follows and a similar need for repeated assessment.

In either of these cases, there may be a decision made for the parents to continue caring for the baby, or there may be a decision for voluntary relinquishment. In the latter case the juvenile court becomes involved to designate a court-appointed advocate for the child and a foster mother to provide care.

The final path in the non-treatment case would usually, though not always, lead to death.

The conference may lead to another outcome: the physicians' advice is rejected. The physician may then find that the duty and interest to care for the child may be sufficiently compelling to continue the professional relationship. In other cases the physician may find the partial caring relationship intolerable and attempt to refer elsewhere for care. In the third alternative, the physician may believe that there is probably cause to believe that refusal for treatment would constitute neglect, or worse, the equivalent of homicide. In this case, the physician would be obliged to confront the issue with the parents and, given their continuing refusal, would need to involve the juvenile court to make a decision as to how the child will be treated. If the court decides in favor of treatment, it will again, as in voluntary relinquishment, appoint an advocate to replace parental responsibility. This does not automatically preclude the continuing parental care, but it may also lead to removal of the infant from the parents and institution of foster care. It is obvious that few physicians would take lightly the violence done to a family in involving them in court action regarding their responsibility, and this last resort is rarely used in practice.

Shurtleff finds that the shock, grief, and confusion of parents of the newborn with congenital malformations, tend to further their dependence on physicians' recommendations. He disagrees with those who believe that parents should bear the final responsibility for making a decision, *since parents may be motivated at times to make a decision against treatment that is contrary to the best interest of the child*. He further believes they should be relieved of the responsibility to initiate a decision to withhold treatment in view of the potential burden of guilt. He advocates that the physician in charge should assume responsibility for making a recommendation to provide ameliorative care only, but should be prepared to choose whether to follow the parents' rejection of his advice in favor of surgical intervention and perform the surgery or to refer the child to a surgeon who will operate. Again, the baby's interest will be well served in the case of quick surgery and discharge from the hospital to the care of a loving mother.

Shurtleff next discusses the treatments available for the various problems and the prognosis in each area. While not engaged in a "list for selection for non-treatment," the tables he and his colleagues have constructed on "Indications for treatment," and "Topics for discussion with parents of patients with myelodysplasia" constitute an excellent framework for physicians and parents to comprehend the nature of the problem, assess prognosis, and make the best decisions they can for the management appropriate to *this infant* [7].

Leonard and Freeman point out that pediatrician advocates must be aware of the advances that have converted spina bifida into a disease entity with 95% survival and a set of manageable problems [17]. This obligation is important to the role of counseling, as well as to assure the multifaceted approach necessary to minimize both disability and handicap. This approach should allow most children the opportunity to be productive adults.

Discussions held with the parents are summarized in written form and are held repeatedly during the long course of the child's care. A pediatrician and nurse are assigned as advocates in each case to coordinate care over the years. Close communication, written and by telephone, is maintained with primary care providers. Shurtleff finds *communication* among the specialists, parents, and primary care providers to be the most essential component of care for the child with chronic handicaps. He recognized the developing increased competence of the family to assimilate information about this complex disorder as it affects their child.

Shurtleff does not feel bound by initial decisions. If, contrary to expectations, an infant thrives, a later back closure and CSF shunt may be performed. If untreatable complications arise as a result of brain destruction from a high-pressure shunt obstruction or CNS infection, an aggressive surgical program may be abandoned.

Parents are given the following assurances:

- The physician will review openly and frequently the progress and prognosis of the child.
- The physician will not recommend treatment for treatment's sake, but only in expectation of benefit to the child.
- The physician will not withhold treatment against the parents' wishes even if there is only a slight chance of success.
- Treatments that will decrease morbidity and relieve suffering will be provided, even if life prolongation is not the goal.
- Increased frequency of review is planned for infants with conditions for whom surgical or medical treatments have been deferred.

Shurtleff concludes by recommending that the physician and other members of the health care team should properly act as an advocate for the child, as well as take responsibility for professional recommendations and actions taken in regard to treatment. He cites that his care program has undergone successful judicial review of decisions, including those leading to nonsurgical treatment and death, and those leading to withdrawal of treatment and death in a child who had initially undergone surgery.

Shurtleff's program is offered as one that appears to fulfill a number of ethical principles. It begins from a base of competence derived from a large experience and a high level of well-trained, intelligent and reflective expertise. It focuses on the patient and its interests at the center of the decision-making process, while it is respectful of the parents—both because their caring attitude is important to the patient and in deference to the considerable needs of the parents who must bear the burden of the care.

Additionally, Shurtleff's program addresses the societal issues. In contrast to a subservient role, the actors in the State of Washington program described by Shurtleff do not seem to deem it their role to protect society from some theoretical burden, but rather count the cost, and work toward the society carrying out its proper role in defense of the fulfilled potential of its handicapped citizens. This appears to be a model of an ethical medical program.

Despite the generally admirable nature of Shurtleff's program certain aspects of the program and its philosophies as described leave some questions needing to be answered.

- Is it really the proper role of the physician to relieve the parents of the decision-making responsibility?
- If the parents are to be primarily responsible for decision-making, to what extent may they be trusted to make these decisions so as to represent the best interest of the child?
- Regardless of the effort to keep the central focus of decision-making the best interest of the child, do Shurtleff's "Indications for treatment" really significantly differ from the use of selective criteria for nontreatment?
- If physicians disagree about the validity of specific selective criteria and ethicists and moral theologians differ widely regarding the appropriateness of various courses of action, how might we better ensure the action that would most appropriately serve the best interests of our patients?
- Finally, what is it about the newborn that apparently engenders a greater motivation to undertake choices among decisions that lead to consequences of life or death?

Jonsen et al. have stated some fundamental ethical propositions as a basis for "a moral policy for newborn intensive care" [18].

1. *Every baby* born possesses a *moral value*, which entitles it to the medical and social care necessary to effect its well-being.

— Moral value indicates that the infant, although unable to comprehend, decide, communicate, or defend its existence, requires by its very existence to be approached with attitudes of respect, consideration, and care. The infant is designated as a being in its own right and morally, if not physically, autonomous. Its life is not merely a function of others.

2. *Parents* bear the principal *moral responsibility* for the well-being of their newborn infant.

— *Responsibility* signifies that those who engender and bring an infant to birth are morally accountable for its well-being. They are closest to the infant and must bear the burdens of its nurture, especially if it is ill or defective. Despite this principle it is recognized that some parents will not or cannot exercise this responsibility. But it states an ideal and a demand which medical professionals should acknowledge in their attitude and in their institutional arrangements.

3. *Physicians* have the *duty* to take medical measures conducive to the well-being of the baby in proportion to their contractual relationships of trust to the parents.

— *Duty* applies to the professional relationships of a physician who has two clients, the infant and the parents. This relationship is fiduciary, that is, a contractual one entered into freely by the physician with the parents who entrust their infant to the medical judgment of the physician for the sake of the infant's well-being. Informed consent *usually* controls fiduciary relationships. However, an infant, the proper patient in this relationship, is unable to be a consenting partner. Thus, parental decisions normally control the relationships. However, the physician responding directly to the moral value of the infant–patient, may at times be duty-bound to resist a parental decision.

The designation of fields of force of parental responsibility and physician's duty means that ultimate decisions, morally, lie with the parents. This does not, in fact, mean that parents will make those decisions always. They may absent themselves physically or psychologically. They may even abdicate their moral right to make decisions by failure to acknowledge the well-being of the infant upon which their responsibility is predicated. In such cases, the duty of the physician is expanded to include the heavy burden of rendering final decisions.

4. The *State* has an *interest* in the proper fulfillment of responsibilities and duties regarding the well-being of the infant.

— *Interest* designates the concern of the State, in particular, and society at large that actions of individuals respect certain values and fulfill certain responsibilities and duties.

Thus, the *value* of the *infant* attracts respect, consideration, and care and repels indifference, violence, and neglect. *Responsibility* attracts specific forms of care for the infant and repels unconcern. The fields of force converge in decisions about neonatal survival, so that the valued infant is the focus of parental responsibility, physician duty, and State interest. Each of these has its limits; each is subordinate to the moral value of the infant.

These principles might seem to imply that withholding of specific therapy would be unethical, since the parents have responsibility to nourish the infant, the physician the duty to cure its illness, and the State has the interest to punish the neglect of the infant. Yet the medical principle "to do no harm" admits of no exceptions, while the moral obligation to "preserve life" is a qualified one. Physicians perform many hurtful acts by necessity; the transient harm is justified by compensating benefits. If no benefit can be reasonably expected, the intervention is unethical. In the context of life conditions that can't be remedied, intensive therapy appears harmful. These conditions are identified as inability to survive a brief period of infancy, inability to live without severe, intractible pain, and inability to participate, at least minimally, in human experience. According to Veatch, in the case of spina bifida treatment, medical intervention may indefinitely extend living, but with a patient-centered burden that some would judge too great [19]. Conservative traditions, such as the Roman Catholic medical-moral theology, recognize some medical treatments as inflicting such a grave burden as to be expendable [19]. Parents, with the responsibility to serve the interests of their child, would be expected to defend their children from excessively burdensome treatments in direct proportion to the degree that they would resist these interventions to themselves. And if a treatment for the child is widely accepted by reasonable people as inflicting grave burden, then society ought to support parents in the treatment refusal decision. It is widely agreed that the physician has no right to intervene against parental wishes, barring an emergency, without a court order [19].

The decision about the care of the abnormal newborn is essentially one which is moral or theological or philosophical. The central decision makers must be those with the moral teaching authority for the child [19]. In some traditions this is a priest or rabbi. For others who believe in the crucial importance of parental responsibility in the care and nurture of the children of a family, the parents must be central no matter how important the physician's values are in dictating his own behavior, unless one is to be seen as taking on the priestly function of determining values for patients. The role should not include making such fateful moral choices as whether or not to operate on an abnormal child. That decision must be made by those responsible for the moral nurture of the child, normally the parents, but the parents placed strictly within the confines of society's judgments of the limits of reasonableness. It is not that the parents have the *right* to decide—rather they have the *obligation* to make such critical choices, until such time as there is reasonable evidence that they are not acting in the interests of the child. In the contract-responsibility model of the roles of the physicians, the parents, and of society, the decision-making process will be a difficult one. It will produce anxiety and ambivalence and agony. But it may also produce responsible human agents contracting together to produce moral medical care. The unattractive alternatives described by Veatch are the physician as priest, or the physician as engineer.

What of selective criteria? Again, according to Veatch, the objection to technical criteria is not only in the vagaries of the precise content of the list. Rather it is the concept that *any* list of objectively measurable criteria can be translated directly into decisions about selection for treatment or non-treatment [19]. The lists appear to be intended to be reasonably accurate measures of prognosis. Yet the presumption that treatment/non-treatment decision rests solely on prognosis is contested. The decision must also include evaluation of the meaning of existence with varying impairments. Great variation exists about these essentially evaluative elements among parents, physicians, and policy makers. When Lorber uses the phrase "contraindications to active therapy," he is seen as medicalizing what are really value choices. (These values are very dependent upon our perceptions. Certain ethicists have discussed "Criteria of Humanhood" [20].)

If non-treatment decisions are assumed to be acceptable it seems plausible that there must be some range of cases for which discretion based on particular sets of religious, cultural, or personal values is appropriate. At the very least parents who want to treat a child who falls within the group of those who have "contraindications for active therapy" should be permitted to act on their moral convictions. Veatch therefore argues that technical measures of prognosis only be a part of the guidelines governing treatment/non-treatment decisions and that families' ethical judgments remain central to the decision-making process, as these are fundamentally quesions of ethical and other values [19].

If technical guidelines vary and are limited in value, if ethicists disagree, and if parents and physicians are limited in their devotion to the interests of the patient and in their competence, then how are we to proceed? My summary answer, based upon experience with a regular frequency of confrontation with agonizing case situations, is simply to state: with greatest humility—open to lots of help.

Norman Fost, a pediatrician-ethicist, proposes a *process* for assisting the family in decision-making [21]. He begins by posting the qualities of the "ideal ethical observor," who would have the following characteristics: (1) *Omniscience*, that is, having all the relevant facts; (2) *Omnipercipience*, having the ability to imagine how others are affected by one's actions; (3) *Disinterestedness*, being impartial, free of self-interest; (4) *Dispassionateness*, free of strong feeling tending to distort judgment; and (5) *Consistency*, using principles which can be applied by others in similar situations. No one and no group of people satisfy the characteristics of the "ideal observor." Parent and physician roles are likely to be specifically limited in some of the qualities.

In the category of *omnisicience*, it is a basic principle that good ethics start with good facts. Among the questionable assertions driving a bias toward non-treatment in myelodysplasia conditions are the suppositions of high probability of a life of misery for the survivors, a high degree of potential for serious family disruption, and the expectations that untreated infants may be confidently expected to quickly die. All of these assertions on close examination have been undocumented and given current capability, prevailing tendencies toward opposite outcomes are possible in most cases.

In *omnipercipience*, the ability to co-feel should incorporate the experience of many adults who have experienced the condition, and consider whether they are not much more accepting than supposed, and also how it affects them to undergo critical procedures in the hands of caretakers who may view them as dismal specimens of limited humanity. Judi Silverstein reports that among young adults with spina bifida the major crippling factor is not the level of the lesion nor the intellectual capacity, but rather the effect of inappropriate attitudes of parents and society [22].

As for *disinterest*, there are varying grounds for conflicts of interests for both parents and physicians. The parents may very understandably feel that prospects of psychological and financial burdens are too much to bear, yet be expected to make decisions on behalf of the best interests of the child. For the physician it is depressing and frustrating to one's motivation to cure to be faced with only the option to care [23].

Dispassionateness is a quality that cannot be expected of parents at all in the initial confrontation with the newborn's defect. On the part of the caretaker, it is most important to avoid emotionally-charged descriptive terms that inappropriately convey either horror or false hope. *Consistency* calls for an attitude that applies similar counsel for non-intervention to patients of all ages with similarly disabling conditions.

Since no one person can possess the idealized qualities of the "ideal observor" and all persons possess a number of identifiable limitations, Fost argues for a *process* that involves other parties. In less formal settings, when faced with conditions posing ethical dilemmas, the prudent physician will involve a consultant for an independent opinion. The family should also be encouraged to involve a trusted family advisor to assist them in clarifying issues and choices. This could be clergy or a respected friend or family member. In major hospital settings the "ideal observor" may be approximated by a multidisciplinary hospital ethics committee. Such a committee would have representatives from medicine, nursing, theology, philosophy, law, and patient advocacy. It would be so composed as to provide competence for consideration of medical facts, and a balanced spectrum of theological and philosophical schools. To represent the particular moral perspective of the involved family, appropriate participants from their persuasion can be included when considering their problem. The role of such a committee is to develop a competence for ethical deliberation and interest analysis. It is to advise and counsel, not to dictate or order actions. Such process can serve a most useful purpose in clarifying the thinking of the principal actors.

In the extreme case, as previously noted, the third party involved in decision-making will be the court [7]. As tragic as this extremity may be, it may be required to fulfill the due process deserts of the immature patient unable to express or order its own desires.

What are the economic considerations in management of myelodysplasia? Again, we are indebted to Shurtleff, who has calculated the cost of providing maximal treatment to 319 spina bifida patients to age six years [24,25]. Patients were grouped by level of lesion and expenditures for maximal care were compared to expenditures made for institutionalized or foster care children.

The advantage expenditures made for the group with lower lumbar or high lumbar lesions were not significantly different for the first 6 years of care, averaging approximately $16,000, while care for sacral level lesions was 36.7% less. Costs for institutional care or foster home care over 3.4 years, at over $17,000, exceeded the mean maximal care expenditures for all patients by approximately 20%. Shurtleff found that costs for support of non-treated survivors were higher, primarily due to abandonment, resulting in higher custodial costs. Increased intellectual and physical impairment among the groups provided with delayed or no surgical treatment probably account for the higher rate of abandonment and resultant higher custodial costs.

Continuing costs throughout life are great after the age of eight years, though the period of significant medical expense has passed. The remaining costs are for brace and wheelchair replacements, annual urological evaluations, and for disposable items. A lifetime bill for disposables can range from $18,000 to $36,000 computed to age sixty. Such items are poorly covered by private insurance or government funding.

It is recommended that counseling in the decision-making process should avoid influencing young parents toward selection for non-treatment on the basis of financial burden [26]. The alternative is to assist the family in mobilizing all available assistance from governmental and voluntary agencies to reduce the financial burden on the family.

The other side of the economic equation is the economic earning power of the handicapped individual. A series reviewed by Gordon, Swinyard, Chambe, and Mesch at New York University in 1978 found that, of 75 patients aged 14 to 37, 52% were attending school, 21% were not in school nor employed, and 27% were employed in competitive industry, the home or sheltered workshops [26]. Another survey found that 69% of traumatic paraplegic patients become employed [27].

If spina bifida patients achieve the goal of self-support, aside from benefits of enhanced personal feelings of self-worth and independence derived from employment, it is found that for every dollar spent on vocational training of a handicapped patient, five dollars are returned by the worker in federal income taxes during the first five years of employment after rehabilitation [28]. If one is concerned with net costs of medical and rehabilitation services for spina bifida patients, the survivors must be given an opportunity to utilize the vocational potential which they have [26].

Success is relative to the environment as well as to the intrinsic status of the individual. So it has been pointed out that a robust 30-year-old man or woman would not be viable if exposed naked at the North Pole. Lee, Jonsen, and Dooley find that parents of children with myelodysplasia must turn to an inadequately funded, fragmented and inequitable system plagued with bureaucratic barriers. They do not find this to be justifiable on the basis of scarce resources [29]. Rather they believe that fragmentation, underfunding and lack of comprehensiveness represent an implicit social consensus about the lack of value of the non-productive, unrehabilitable and "different" members of society. They advocate that societal programs should seek to improve the lives of the disabled, regardless of whether or not the improvements involve an economic return for society.

A family deciding about the care of a child with myelodysplasia will reflect their own psychological and social ability to deal with that child. They should be free to look primarily at the child, his/her possibilities and at their own human strengths and weaknesses. Their decisions should not have to be burdened by the economics of the child's care or on bureaucratic complexities in obtaining the funding for care.

When parents consider the quality of life for their child, they join society in looking with horror upon the prospect of a life on welfare, with little prospect of a rewarding job, future family, a decent standard of living, and the continued stigma of being different. These are values enforced by an intolerant society.

The authors maintain that there are little data to support the contention that resources are too scarce to adequately support the handicapped. They maintain that as best that can be judged on the basis of limited data available, anticipated costs for optimal care for the handicapped will not lay an unfair or disproportionate burden on American society. They call for programs designed to place functional competence at equal stature with economic competence as a goal. Fragmentation should be eliminated and comprehensiveness improved.

If it becomes clear that costs of providing optimal medical and social care for severely damaged children has become so expensive that other crucial social programs are damaged, it will then be necessary to make hard judgments about priorities. That time has not arrived. The societal values relating to the disabled have yet to be acknowledged. The time has come for both values and policies to be examined.

Impairment is the amount of fixed deficit, while handicap is the disability superimposed on that deficit by society. As physicians we should remind ourselves that research in improved medical care, development of innovative techniques and reorientation of public attitudes towards the handicapped will improve the quality of life in store for these children. Advances in medical care are not made by turning our backs on the difficult problems.

In closing, I must ask the questions, why does it seem relatively easier, albeit with sorrow, for us to face hard choices, when we contemplate the newborn with severe defects? Do we really as readily face these issues in the other segments of our lifespan? I suspect not. I can only speculate why this might be true. I would then consider that the newborn has no voice, no competence to decide its own fate, no vote, and no economic value. I would also note that we are very much taken up with our individuality, our freedom, our power. The newborn represents responsibility and a sure change in the lifestyle of its parents.

Perhaps there are some attributes in our psyche attached to the newborn that are more subtle. The ethicist and theologian, John Fletcher, offers to us some insight [30].

The profound grief on the birth of a seriously defective infant can be better understood if one considers the symbolic impact of a "ruined natality event." Hannah Arendt has eloquently argued that two of the basic conditions of human life, action and work, are deeply rooted in the birth events of mankind [31]. Natality events, in every culture, are the focus for hope that the laws of mortality and the cycle of the biological process are not the final comments on the meaning of human existence.

The miracle that saves the world, the realm of human affairs, from its normal, "natural" ruin is ultimately the fact of natality, in which the faculty of action is originally rooted. It is, in other words, the birth of new men and women and the new beginning, the action they are capable of by virtue of being born. Only the full experience of this capacity can bestow upon human affairs faith and hope.

Robert Jay Lifton's studies of symbolic immortality" include the event of childbirth as one in which a mode of immortality, "experiential transcendence," may occur in which people transcend the ordinary limits of time and daily life [32]. The biological process of pregnancy prepared the parents, especially the mother, for the appearance of a unique individual. It would seem that all of the cultural and biological systems of humans work together to prepare for the child who appears with the force of a miracle, or at least as the center of an event that has the capacity to elevate parents and their helpers beyond the cloying downward pull of the everyday.

And what happens when, through no intentionality of their own, the child presents itself with a serious disease, even one that defies therapy? The initial, universally negative reaction to the defective newborn unites all participants in confrontation with the terror of death even in the sublime moment of birth. At the initial level, nothing is expected but a negative response to the seriously defective newborn. It is in the second layer of response, when the different authority and reference groups to which all respond, come into play, that the attitudes described begin to function. After the initial shock has passed, it is known that the decisions must be made with the possibilities and limits that training, ethics, and circumstances make available. The profound ambivalence towards the defective newborn might be understood in the context of the struggle with the tension between a primitive/emotive response to be rid of the infant (because of the anxiety it creates) and a second, more socialized response to behave as one believes one ought to have in caring for the infant.

Those who experience this profound ambivalance in varying ways have their unity in the common human experience of external disruption of the normal repression of the terror of death and one's own mortality.

How beautiful and terrible is this scenario. What an enormous burden is the baggage the newborn brings with it as it emerges into our society. I would like to close with the beauty of James Agee's poetry:

> I have been fashioned on a chain of flesh whose ancient lengths lie immolate in dust; Frail though that dust be as the dew's mesh the morning mars, it holds me to a trust. (James Agee, *Permit Me Voyage*, 1934.)

and

> In each child who is born under no matter what circumstances, and of no matter what parents, the potentiality of the human race is born again: and in him too, once more, and of each of us, our terrific responsibility towards human life; towards the utmost idea of goodness, of the horror of error, and of God. (James Agee, *Let Us Now Praise Famous Men*, 1941.)

REFERENCES

1. Swinyard, C. A. *Decision Making and the Defective Newborn*. Springfield, Ill.: Charles C Thomas Co., 1978.
2. Combe, A. *A Treatise on the Physiological and Moral Management of Infancy, for the Use of Parents*, 4th ed. New York: William H. Colyer, 1845.

 3. Rickham, P. P. The ethics of surgery in newborn infants. In: *Neonatal Surgery*, edited by P. P. Rickham and J. H. Johnston. New York: Appleton-Century-Crofts, 1969.
 4. Daily, W. J. R. Personal communication.
 5. Halpe, P. R., Daily, W. J. R., Meyer, H. B. P., and Hart, M. C. Altered prognosis for babies <1500 grams who need mechanical ventilation. *Clin. Res. 23*:158A, 1975.
 6. Sell, E. J. Follow-up of the Infant Given Neonatal Intensive Care. Presented at the *Barrows Institute Annual Symposium*, February, 1983.
 7. Shurtleff, D. B. Myelodysplasia: management and treatment. *Curr. Probl. Pediatr. 10*:3, 1980.
 8. Bakan, D. *Slaughter of the Innocents*. San Francisco: Jossey Bass, 1971.
 9. Wertham, F. *A Sign for Cain: An Exploration of Human Violence*. New York: MacMillian, 1962.
10. Menelans, M. E. *The Orthopedic Management of Spina Bifida Cystica*. Edinburgh: Livingston, 1971.
11. Veatch, R. M. The technical criteria fallacy. *Hastings Cent. Rep. 7*:15–16, 1977.
12. Rickham, P. P. The swing of the pendulum: The indications for operating on meningomyelocele. *Med. J. Aust. 2*:743, 1976.
13. Robardo, M. F., Thomas, G. G., and Rosenbloom, L. Survival of infants with unoperated myeloceles. *Br. Med. J. 4*:12, 1975.
14. Shurtleff, D. B., et al. Myelodysplasia: Decision for death or disability. *N. Engl. J. Med. 291*:1005, 1974.
15. DeLange, S. A. Selection for treatment of patients with spina bifida operta. *Dev. Med. Child. Neurol. 16*(suppl. 32):27, 1974.
16. Freeman, J. M. The shortsighted treatment of meningomyelocele: A long-term case report. *Pediatrics 53*:311, 1974.
17. Leonard, C. E., and Freeman, J. M. Spina bifida: a new disease. *Pediatrics 68*:136, 1981.
18. Jonsen, A. R., Phibbs, R. H., Tooley, W. H., and Garland, M. J. Critical issues in newborn intensive care: A conference report and policy proposal. *Pediatrics 55*:756, 1975.
19. Veatch, R. M. Abnormal newborns and the physician's role: models of physician decision making. In: *Decision Making and the Defective Newborn*, editied by C. A. Swinyard. Spiringfield, Ill: Charles C Thomas, 1978.
20. Fletcher, J. Four indications of humanhood: The enquiry matures. *Hastings Cent. Rep. 4*:4, 1974.
21. Fost, N. How decisions are made: A physician's view. In: *Decision Making and the Defective Newborn*, edited by C. A. Swinyard. Springfield, Ill.: Charles C Thomas, 1978.
22. Silverstein, J. Discussion. In: *Decision Making and the Defective Newborn*, edited by C. A. Swinyard. Springfield, Ill.: Charles C Thomas, 1978.
23. Darling, R. B. Parents, physicians, and spina bifida. *Hastings Cent. Rep. 7*:10, 1977.
24. Shurtleff, D. B., and Lamers, J. Clinical considerations in the treatment of myelodysplasia. In: *Prevention of Neural Tube Defects: The Role of Alpha-feto Protein*, edited by B. F. Crandall and M. A. B. Brazier. New York: Academic Press, 1978.

25. Shurtleff, D. B., et al. Myelodysplasia: decision for death or disability. *N. Engl. J. Med. 291*:1005, 1974.
26. Gordon, W. A., Swinyard, C. A., Chaube, S., and Mesch, J. Economic aspects of spina bifida care. In: *Decision Making and the Defective Newborn*, edited by C. A. Swinyard. Springfield, Ill.: Charles C Thomas, 1978.
27. Guttman, L. Statistical survey on one thousand paraplegics and initial treatment of traumatic paraplegia. *Proc. R. Soc. Med. 47*:1009, 1954.
28. Rusk, H. A. *Rehabilitation Medicine*, 3rd ed. St. Louis: C. V. Mosby, Co., 1971.
29. Lee, P. R., Jonsen, A. R., and Dooley, D. Social and economic factors affecting public policy and decision making in the care of the defective newborn. In: *Decision Making and the Defective Newborn*, edited by C. A. Swinyard. Springfield, Ill.: Charles C Thomas, 1978.
30. Fletcher, J. Spina bifida with meningomyelocele: A case study in attitudes towards defective newborns. In: *Decision Making and the Defective Newborn*, edited by C. A. Swinyard. Springfield, Ill.: Charles C Thomas, 1978.
31. Arendt, H. *The Human Condition*. Chicago: University of Chicago Press, 1959.
32. Lifton, R. J., and Olson, E. *Living and Dying*. New York: Praeger, 1974.

Index

Acidosis, 28
Agee, James, 209
Agenesis of corpus callosum, 73
Alert state of consciousness, 151
Alobar holoprosencephaly, 73
Amniotic fluid, 5, 6
Amplitude ratio (AR), 92-94
Anencephaly, 115
Anoxemia, 28
Antibiotic prophylaxis for
     myelomeningocele, 122-
     123
Apgar score, 147
Apnea
   abnormal, 129
   clinical syndromes, 133-134
   consequences of, 130-132
   noisy breathing with structural
     defect, 135
   noisy breathing without structural
     defect, 136
   normal, 129
   obstructive syndrome, 140-141
   silent with neurological signs, 134
   silent without neurological signs,
     135
   sleep and, 132-133
AR (amplitude ratio), 92-94
Arachnoid cyst, 72
Arendt, Hannah, 208
Arnold-Chiari malformation, 73, 116,
     124
Arteriovenous malformations, 74
Asphyxia, 17, 24, 46
   neonatorum, 57-63
     diagnosis of, 61

[Asphyxia]
   partial, 26, 28
   prolonged partial, 26
   total, 28
Assessment, neurological, see Neuro-
     logical assessment, clinical,
     of neonate
Astrocytosis, 24
Auditory-evoked potentials, see Brain-
     stem auditory-evoked
     potentials
Autoregulation, 48
   loss of, 45

Barium, injection of, 45
Birthweight
   very low (VLBW), 168-172
   very, very low (VVLBW), 169-172
Biventricular cardiac failure, 140
Blood-brain barrier, hypoxic-ischemic
     damage to, 34
Blood flow, cerebral, see Cerebral
     blood flow
BNBAS (Brazelton Neonatal Behavioral
     Assessment Scale), 173, 174
BPD (bronchopulmonary dysplasia),
     172-179
Brain
   noncystic malformations of, 73-74
   prenatal development of, 1
Brain capillaries, 149
Brain damage
   distribution of, 26, 28
   hypoxic-ischemic, see Hypoxic-
     ischemic brain damage
Brain edema, 26

213